SALADS FOR DIABETICS AND DIETERS

SALADS FOR DIABETICS
AND DIETERS

SUZANNE BINET

GAGE PUBLISHING
TORONTO • VANCOUVER • CALGARY • MONTREAL

Cover Photo: Shin Sugino

Canadian Cataloguing in Publication Data

Binet, Suzanne, 1952 —
Salads for diabetics and dieters

Translation of Salades — santé.

ISBN 0-7715-9487-9

1. Cookery for diabetics.   2. Salads.
I. Title

RC662.B5613   641.8'3   C79-09416501

1 2 3 4 HR 82 81 80 79

Printed and bound in Canada.

Foreword

A salad! What could be more simple yet more sophisticated at the same time? You do not have to wait for the first fruits of the summer to treat yourselves; the fruits and vegetables needed for a salad's preparation are available all year long. And if you had not thought of salads as a year-round treat before, the recipes contained within should change your mind.

"I am not a vegetarian," you will probably think to yourself. But that is no reason to avoid salads. I am not a vegetarian either, and in my book I show that this is no obstacle to enjoying a salad's varied charms. A salad can be much more than a simple green leaf capriciously enhanced by a dollop of dressing!

The recipes I chose will allow you to elaborate on a simple menu or to complete it with a special touch. Finally, the choice is yours, whether you want a salad entrée, a meal, a dessert or just a nice, little salad.

A very good friend of mine told me in confidence that he never spent a day without eating his bowl of soup and his salad. A fanatic? Not at all! Soup warms the heart and salad gives you freshness, color and all sorts of other good things, which I invite you to discover. Only taste some of the recipes in here and I'm sure you will agree with me.

Suzanne Binet

Vegetable Salads

Asparagus from Russia

Ingredients:	Wt.	C	P	F
35 fresh asparagus spears, cooked, cooled and cut in 2" pieces (5 cm)	420g	35	7	–
4 cups lettuce leaves, torn	280g	20	4	–
1 cup celery, thinly sliced	128g	2.5	.5	–
1 small onion, minced	35g	5	1	–
5 tsp. salad oil	25g	–	–	25
2 tbsp. vinegar	30g	–	–	–
2 tbsp. fresh lemon juice	25g	2.5	–	–
1/4 cup cooked beets, chopped	38g	5	.5	–
1 hard-cooked egg, chopped	50g	–	7	5
1 tbsp. snipped parsley	3.5g	–	–	–
1 tsp. paprika	5g	–	–	–
1 tsp. sugar	5g	5	.6	–
1 tsp. salt	5g	–	–	–
1/2 tsp. dry mustard	2.5g	–	–	–
1/4 tsp. Worcestershire sauce	–	–	–	–

Preparation: Combine asparagus, lettuce, celery and onion. In a jar with lid, combine rest of ingredients; cover and shake well. Pour this dressing over salad and toss slightly until each piece is shining.

Calories: 652 or 109 calories/serving

Servings: 6

Exchange Value:

1/2 bread exchange +
1 5% vegetable exchange +
1 fat exchange

or

1 10% vegetable exchange +
1/2 fat exchange +
1/4 whole milk exchange (2 ounces)

or

1/2 meat exchange +
1 10% vegetable exchange +
1/2 fat exchange

Beans and Cabbage Salad

Ingredients:	Wt.	C	P	F
3 bacon slices	30g	–	7	5
2 tbsp. bacon fat	30g	–	–	30
1 small onion, minced	35g	5	1	–
1/4 cup wine vinegar	60g	–	–	–
1 tsp. sugar	5g	5	.6	–
1/2 tsp. salt	2.5g	–	–	–
dash pepper	–	–	–	–
2 cups raw cabbage, shredded	200g	20	4	–
2 cups small Lima beans, cooked	330g	90	12	–

Preparation: In a small skillet, fry bacon until crisp; drain, keeping only 2 tbsp. bacon fat. Crumble bacon and set aside. Cook onion in bacon fat until golden brown; add vinegar, sugar, salt and pepper. Let simmer a few minutes, then pour mixture over combined cabbage and beans. Toss well and sprinkle with crumbled bacon.

Calories: 894 or 149 calories/serving
Servings: 6
Exchange Value:

1 1/2 bread exchange +
1 fat exchange
           or
1/2 bread exchange +
1 5% vegetable exchange +
1/2 whole milk exchange (4 ounces)

Corn Picnic

Ingredients:	Wt.	C	P	F
1 1/3 cups whole kernel corn	300g	60	8	–
1 medium cucumber, unpeeled and diced	100g	10	2	–
1/4 tsp. onion powder	–	–	–	–
4 bacon slices, crisp, drained, and crumbled	40g	–	–	20
1 tbsp. vinegar	15g	–	–	–
1/4 tsp. paprika	–	–	–	–
1/4 tsp. Worcestershire sauce	–	–	–	–
1/4 tsp. salt	–	–	–	–

Preparation: Combine all ingredients; toss lightly and refrigerate.

Calories: 500 or 125 calories/serving
Servings: 4
Exchange Value:
1/2 bread exchange +
1 10% vegetable exchange +
1 fat exchange

Creamed Lettuce

Ingredients:	Wt.	C	P	F
1/2 cup light cream (15%)	120g	–	–	20
1 tsp. sugar	5g	5	.6	–
1/4 cup vinegar	60g	–	–	–
1/4 tsp. salt	–	–	–	–
4 cups lettuce leaves, torn	280g	20	4	–
1 scallion, minced	20g	–	–	–

Preparation: Mix the first 4 ingredients well. Combine lettuce and scallion in a salad bowl; drizzle with dressing and toss lightly. Serve immediately.

Calories: 298 or 75 calories/serving

Servings: 4

Exchange Value: 1/2 bread exchange +
1 fat exchange

Crisp Bacon and Tomato Salad

Ingredients:	Wt.	C	P	F
2 bread slices	60g	30	4	–
3 cups lettuce leaves, torn	210g	15	3	–
3 medium tomatoes, sliced in small quarters	270g	15	3	–
6 bacon slices, crisp, drained and crumbled	60g	–	14	10
3 ounces or 6 tbsp. dietetic mayonnaise	90g	–	–	10

Preparation: Cut bread slices in ½" (1.25 cm) cubes and let dry in a preheated oven (225°F or 107°C), about 2 hours. Line salad bowl with lettuce leaves. In the same bowl, combine bread cubes, torn lettuce leaves, tomatoes, bacon and mayonnaise. Toss lightly and season to taste.

Calories: 516 or 129 calories/serving

Servings: 4

Exchange Value:
½ meat exchange +
1 bread exchange +
½ fat exchange
           or
1 fruit exchange +
½ whole milk exchange (4 ounces)

Enhanced Spinach Salad

Ingredients:	Wt.	C	P	F
3 bacon slices	30g	–	7	5
1 tbsp. bacon fat	15g	–	–	15
1/4 cup vinegar	60g	–	–	–
2 tsp. salad oil	10g	–	–	10
1 1/2 tsp. sugar	7.5g	7.5	1	–
1/4 tsp. salt	–	–	–	–
dash pepper	–	–	–	–
1/2 small scallion, minced	10g	–	–	–
6 cups spinach leaves, torn	420g	30	6	–

Preparation: In a large skillet, cook bacon slices until crisp; drain, keeping only 1 tbsp. bacon fat. Crumble bacon and set aside. Add vinegar, oil, sugar, salt and pepper to bacon fat. Bring to boil and add scallion. Gradually, add spinach leaves; toss lightly, just until each piece is coated with dressing. Sprinkle with crumbled bacon.

Calories: 476 or 79 calories/serving

Servings: 6

Exchange Value: 1/2 bread exchange + 1 fat exchange

Fresh Salad

Ingredients:	Wt.	C	P	F
3 medium cucumbers, unpeeled and thinly sliced	300g	30	6	–
1 tsp. salt	5g	–	–	–
1 small scallion, minced	20g	–	–	–
1 tbsp. salad oil	15g	–	–	15
1 tbsp. vinegar	15g	–	–	–
1 tsp. sugar	5g	5	.6	–
dash pepper	–	–	–	–

Preparation: Place cucumber slices in a large bowl; sprinkle with salt. Cover and let steep 1 hour. Drain well and add scallion. Mix rest of ingredients in a small saucepan; bring to boiling point and pour over cucumber slices. Refrigerate.

Calories: 301 or 50 calories/serving
Servings: 6
Exchange Value: 1 5% vegetable exchange + $1/2$ fat exchange

Green Leaves "Extra"

Ingredients:	Wt.	C	P	F
3 bacon slices, diced	30g	–	–	15
1 tbsp. bacon fat	15g	–	–	15
3 cups lettuce leaves, torn	210g	15	3	–
3 cups spinach leaves, torn	210g	15	3	–
1/2 cup celery, diced	64g	–	–	–
1 ounce or 1/4 cup blue Danish cheese	30g	–	7	5
1/2 small scallion, minced	10g	–	–	–
1/4 cup vinegar	60g	–	–	–
2 tbsp. sugar	30g	30	4	–
1/2 tsp. Worcestershire sauce	2.5g	–	–	–

Preparation: In a small skillet, cook bacon slices until crisp; drain, keeping only 1 tbsp. bacon fat. Crumble bacon and set aside. In a large salad bowl, combine lettuce and spinach leaves, bacon, celery, cheese and scallion. Add vinegar, sugar and Worcestershire sauce to bacon fat; bring to boil. Pour over salad and toss carefully.

Calories: 623 or 104 calories/serving

Servings: 6

Exchange Value:

1/2 bread exchange +
1/2 fat exchange +
1/4 whole milk exchange (2 ounces)
                    or
1/2 meat exchange +
1 fruit exchange +
1/2 fat exchange

"King of Garden" Salad

Ingredients:	Wt.	C	P	F
2 medium cucumbers, unpeeled and thinly sliced	200g	20	4	–
1/2 cup dairy sour cream	120g	–	–	20
1 tbsp. lemon juice	12g	–	–	–
1/2 tsp. salt	2.5g	–	–	–
1/8 tsp. dry mustard	–	–	–	–

Preparation: Mix sour cream, lemon juice, salt and mustard well. Pour over cucumber slices and toss. Refrigerate. Serve on lettuce leaves.

Calories: 276 or 69 calories/serving
Servings: 4
Exchange Value: 1 5% vegetable exchange + 1 fat exchange

Luigi Lima Beans

Ingredients:	Wt.	C	P	F
1 1/3 cups small Lima beans, cooked and well cooled	320g	60	8	–
1/4 cup dairy sour cream	60g	–	–	10
1 tbsp. vinegar	15g	–	–	–
1 small clove garlic, minced	–	–	–	–
1/2 tsp. sugar	2.5g	2.5	–	–
1/4 tsp. salt	–	–	–	–
dash paprika	–	–	–	–

Preparation: Mix sour cream, vinegar, garlic, sugar, salt and paprika well. Add Lima beans and toss until each piece is well moistened. Serve on lettuce.

Calories: 372 or 93 calories/serving
Servings: 4
Exchange Value: 1 bread exchange + 1/2 fat exchange

Nautical Cucumbers

Ingredients:	Wt.	C	P	F
2 medium cucumbers	200g	20	4	–
10 medium shrimps, cooked and cleaned	60g	–	14	10
1/4 cup vinegar	60g	–	–	–
1 tbsp. sugar	15g	15	2	–
1/2 tsp. soya sauce	2.5g	–	–	–
1/2 tsp. salt	2.5g	–	–	–

Preparation: Peel cucumbers and slice 1/4" (.625 cm) thin. Place in a medium bowl and add shrimps. Mix vinegar, sugar, soya sauce and salt; pour over salad. Toss, cover and refrigerate. Drain and serve on lettuce leaves.

Calories: 310 or 78 calories/serving
Servings: 4
Exchange Value: 1/2 meat exchange +
1 10% vegetable exchange

Saucy Spinach

Ingredients:	Wt.	C	P	F
2 cups raw spinach, torn in small pieces	140g	10	2	—
2 scallions, minced	35g	5	1	—
1 medium cucumber, peeled and thinly sliced	100g	10	2	—
salt and pepper to taste	—	—	—	—
2 cups cottage cheese (creamed)	480g	—	56	40
1 cup dairy sour cream	240g	—	—	40
2 tsp. lemon juice	8g	—	—	—

Preparation: Toss together the first 3 ingredients; season to taste. Divide salad and place in individual bowls; put 1/2 cup cottage cheese in centre of each salad bowl. Combine sour cream and lemon juice and mix well; pour 1/4 cup of this dressing over each serving.

Calories: 1064 or 266 calories/serving

Servings: 4

Exchange Value:

2 meat exchanges +
1/2 bread exchange +
2 fat exchanges
         or
1 1/2 meat exchanges +
1 1/2 fat exchanges +
1/2 whole milk exchange (4 ounces)

Simple Green Salad

Ingredients:	Wt.	C	P	F
1 clove of garlic, sliced	—	—	—	—
1/2 tsp. salt	2.5g	—	—	—
1/4 tsp. dry mustard	—	—	—	—
1/4 tsp. paprika	—	—	—	—
dash pepper	—	—	—	—
4 tsp. salad oil	20g	—	—	20
4 cups green leaves (your choice) torn	280g	20	4	—
2 tbsp. vinegar	30g	—	—	—
2 tbsp. fresh lemon juice	25g	2.5	—	—

Preparation: Rub salad bowl with sliced garlic. In the bottom of the bowl, combine salt, mustard, paprika and pepper; mix well, then add salad oil and beat with a fork. Add green leaves and toss until each piece of salad is shining. Drizzle with vinegar and lemon juice and toss once more.

Calories: 286 or 72 calories/serving

Servings: 4

Exchange Value: 1 5% vegetable exchange +
1 fat exchange

Spinach "Grand-père"

Ingredients:	Wt.	C	P	F
½ small scallion, minced	10g	–	–	–
2 tbsp. butter or margarine	30g	–	–	30
2 tbsp. all-purpose flour	14g	12	1.6	–
dash salt	–	–	–	–
1 cup water	200g	–	–	–
2 tbsp. lemon juice	25g	2	–	–
½ tbsp. horseradish	7.5g	–	–	–
½ tsp. Worcestershire sauce	2.5g	–	–	–
6 cups spinach leaves, torn	420g	30	6	–

Preparation: In a small skillet, make sauce: cook scallion in fat, about 1 minute, then add flour and salt, stirring constantly. Add water, lemon juice, horseradish and Worcestershire sauce. Remove from heat. Put spinach leaves in a large salad bowl and pour hot dressing over. Toss carefully and serve immediately.

Calories: 476 or 79 calories/serving
Servings: 6
Exchange Value: ½ bread exchange + 1 fat exchange

Vegetable Medley

Ingredients:	Wt.	C	P	F
1 cup dairy sour cream	240g	–	–	40
2 tbsp. lemon juice	25g	2.5	–	–
2 tbsp. cider vinegar	30g	–	–	–
2 tbsp. sugar	30g	30	4	–
1 tsp. salt	5g	–	–	–
dash pepper	–	–	–	–
1 tsp. dry mustard	5g	–	–	–
1 cup chopped celery	128g	2.5	.5	–
2 cups raw cabbage, grated	200g	20	4	–
1 medium raw carrot, peeled and grated	88g	10	1	–
1/4 cup raisins	30g	20	2	–

Preparation: Combine the first 7 ingredients and beat until smooth. Add rest of ingredients and toss.

Calories: 746 or 93 calories/serving
Servings: 8
Exchange Value: 1 10% vegetable exchange +
1 fat exchange

Wax Beans Special

Ingredients:	Wt.	C	P	F
2 tbsp. dairy sour cream	30g	–	–	5
1/4 tsp. Worcestershire sauce	–	–	–	–
1 tbsp. cider vinegar	15g	–	–	–
1 tbsp. catsup	15g	–	–	–
1/4 tsp. salt	–	–	–	–
dash pepper	–	–	–	–
4 cups cooked wax beans, cooled and cut in 3/4" pieces (1.875 cm)	600g	40	8	–
minced parsley to taste	–	–	–	–

Preparation: Mix together sour cream, Worcestershire sauce, vinegar, catsup, salt and pepper. Pour this dressing over beans and toss lightly. Marinate in refrigerator at least 1 hour, stirring occasionally. Sprinkle with parsley, if desired. Refrigerate until time to use.

Calories: 237 or 40 calories/serving
Servings: 6
Exchange Value: 1/2 bread exchange

Vegetable Molded Salads

Emergency Salad

Ingredients:	Wt.	C	P	F
1 envelope unflavored gelatin	8g	–	–	–
1 cup cold water, divided	200g	–	–	–
1 can (10½ ounces) cream of celery, undiluted	300g	22.5	3	15
1 tbsp. lemon juice	12g	–	–	–
dash pepper	–	–	–	–
1½ cups cold pressed meat (luncheon meat), diced	270g	–	42	30
½ cup celery, chopped	64g	–	–	–
3 tbsp. pimiento, chopped	45g	–	–	–
½ tsp. onion powder	2.5g	–	–	–

Preparation: In a medium saucepan, soften gelatin in ½ cup cold water. Heat over low heat, stirring constantly, until well dissolved. Remove from heat; add soup and mix well. Add the other ½ cup cold water, lemon juice and pepper. Refrigerate until partially set; fold in meat, celery, pimiento and onion powder. Pour into a 4-cup mold. Refrigerate until set.

Calories: 675 or 169 calories/serving

Servings: 4

Exchange Value:

1½ meat exchanges +
1 5% vegetable exchange +
1 fat exchange

or

1 meat exchange +
½ whole milk exchange (4 ounces)

Molded Coleslaw

Ingredients:	Wt.	C	P	F
1 package (3 ounces) lime flavored gelatin	85g	90	12	—
1/2 tsp. salt	2.5g	—	—	—
1 cup boiling water	200g	—	—	—
2 tbsp. vinegar	30g	—	—	—
1/2 cup cold water	100g	—	—	—
2 cups raw cabbage, shredded	200g	20	4	—
3 ounces or 6 tbsp. dietetic mayonnaise	90g	—	—	10
1/2 cup dairy sour cream	120g	—	—	20
3 tbsp. pimiento, chopped	45g	5	1	—
1 tbsp. prepared mustard	15g	—	—	—
1 tsp. sugar	5g	5	.6	—
1 small scallion, minced	20g	—	—	—

Preparation: Dissolve gelatin and salt in boiling water; add vinegar and cold water. Mix well. Add rest of ingredients and refrigerate until partially set. Mix again and pour into 6 individual molds. Refrigerate until set.

Calories: 820 or 137 calories/serving

Servings: 6

Exchange Value:
1 bread exchange +
1 5% vegetable exchange +
1 fat exchange

Nice Little Vegetable Molds

Ingredients:	Wt.	C	P	F
1 package (3 ounces) lemon flavored gelatin	85g	90	12	—
2 tsp. instant beef broth powder or liquid	10g	—	—	—
1 cup boiling water	200g	—	—	—
3/4 cup dairy sour cream	180g	—	—	30
2 tbsp. vinegar	30g	—	—	—
1/2 cup celery, chopped	64g	—	—	—
1/2 medium cucumber, unpeeled, chopped	50g	5	1	—
1/2 small scallion, minced	10g	—	—	—

Preparation: Dissolve gelatin and beef powder in boiling water. Refrigerate until partially set. Add sour cream and vinegar; beat until very smooth. Fold in rest of ingredients and pour into 6 1/2-cup molds. Refrigerate until set.

Calories: 702 or 117 calories/serving

Servings: 6

Exchange Value:
1 bread exchange
1 fat exchange

Summertime Asparagus

Ingredients:	Wt.	C	P	F
1 envelope unflavored gelatin	8g	–	–	–
1 can (10½ ounces) cream of asparagus, undiluted	300g	22.5	3	7.5
2 tsp. lemon juice	8g	–	–	–
dash salt	–	–	–	–
1 cup creamed cottage cheese	240g	–	28	20
½ cup dairy sour cream	120g	–	–	20
½ cup celery, chopped	64g	–	–	–
1 tbsp. pimiento, chopped	15g	–	–	–

Preparation: In a medium casserole, soften gelatin in ¼ cup cold water. Heat over low heat, stirring constantly, until dissolved. Mix soup, lemon juice and salt well with gelatin; fold in cottage cheese and sour cream. Refrigerate until partially set, then fold in celery and pimiento. Pour into a 4½-cup mold. Refrigerate until set.

Calories: 642 or 107 calories/serving

Servings: 6

Exchange Value:

½ meat exchange +
½ fat exchange +
½ whole milk exchange (2 ounces)
    or
½ meat exchange +
1 5% vegetable exchange +
1 fat exchange

Tomato Mousse

Ingredients:	Wt.	C	P	F
³/₄ cup evaporated milk, very cold	180g	18	12	15
3 cups tomato juice	660g	30	3	–
2 bay leaves	–	–	–	–
¹/₂ tsp. onion salt	2.5g	–	–	–
dash celery salt	–	–	–	–
2 envelopes unflavored gelatin	16g	–	–	–
2 packages (3 ounces each) cream cheese, softened	180g	–	–	60

Preparation: In a large casserole, combine 2 cups tomato juice, bay leaves, onion salt and celery salt. Heat, cover and simmer 5 minutes; remove bay leaves. Soak gelatin in ¹/₂ cup tomato juice; add to hot mixture, stirring until dissolved. Let cool. With an electric mixer, beat cream cheese with rest of tomato juice until mixture is very smooth; add to gelatin mixture. Refrigerate until partially set. Whip evaporated milk until it forms firm peaks; fold into gelatin mixture. Pour into a 6¹/₂-cup mold. Refrigerate until firm.

Calories: 927 or 93 calories/serving
Servings: 10
Exchange Value: 1 5% vegetable exchange +
1¹/₂ fat exchanges

Coleslaws

"Chef" Relish

Ingredients:	Wt.	C	P	F
1 tsp. salt	5g	–	–	–
1/4 tsp. pepper	–	–	–	–
1/2 tsp. dry mustard	2.5g	–	–	–
1/2 tsp. celery salt	2.5g	–	–	–
2 tbsp. sugar	30g	30	4	–
1 tbsp. pimiento, chopped	15g	–	–	–
1 tsp. onion, grated	5g	–	–	–
1/2 cup vinegar	120g	–	–	–
3 cups raw cabbage, shredded	300g	30	6	–

Preparation: Combine all ingredients in a salad bowl and mix well. Refrigerate.

Calories: 280 or 70 calories/serving
Servings: 4
Exchange Value: 1 bread exchange

Coleslaw

Ingredients:	Wt.	C	P	F
2 cups raw cabbage, shredded	200g	20	4	—
2 scallions, minced	35g	5	1	—
2 tbsp. snipped parsley	7g	—	—	—
2 tbsp. sugar	30g	30	4	—
3 tbsp. vinegar	45g	—	—	—
2 tbsp. salad oil	30g	—	—	30
1 tsp. salt	5g	—	—	—

Preparation: Combine cabbage, scallions and parsley; refrigerate. Mix together sugar, vinegar, oil and salt, stirring until sugar is dissolved; refrigerate. Pour vinegar mixture over salad and toss slightly.

Calories: 526 or 88 calories/serving
Servings: 6
Exchange Value: 1 10% vegetable exchange +
1 fat exchange

Coleslaw, Danish Style

Ingredients:	Wt.	C	P	F
6 cups raw cabbage, shredded	600g	60	12	–
1/2 tsp. salt	2.5g	–	–	–
1 tsp. dry mustard	5g	–	–	–
2 tsp. sugar	10g	10	1.2	–
2 1/2 tbsp. flour	18g	15	2	–
1 egg	50g	–	7	5
2 tbsp. butter or margarine	30g	–	–	30
3/4 cup milk	180g	9	6	7.5
1/4 cup cider vinegar	60g	–	–	–

Preparation: Cook cabbage in salted, boiling water until tender but still crisp. Combine salt, mustard, sugar, flour and egg; beat well. Melt fat in the upper part of a double boiler, over very hot water. Add egg mixture and milk; slowly pour in vinegar, stirring constantly, and cook until sauce is smooth and thickened. Pour over cabbage and toss well. Serve in preheated bowls.

Calories: 872 or 145 calories/serving

Servings: 6

Exchange Value:

1/2 meat exchange +
1 bread exchange +
1 fat exchange

Confetti Coleslaw

Ingredients:	Wt.	C	P	F
4 cups raw cabbage, shredded	400g	40	8	—
1 1/3 cups whole kernel corn, cooked	300g	60	8	—
1 medium onion, minced	70g	10	1	—
3 tbsp. pimiento, chopped	45g	5	1	—
1/2 tsp. salt	2.5g	—	—	—
9 tbsp. dietetic mayonnaise	135g	—	—	15

Preparation: Combine the first 4 ingredients; refrigerate. Just before serving, add salt and mayonnaise; toss lightly.

Calories: 667 or 111 calories/serving

Servings: 6

Exchange Value:

1 bread exchange +
1 5% vegetable exchange +
1/2 fat exchange
    or
1 bread exchange +
1/4 whole milk exchange (2 ounces)

Gardener Coleslaw

Ingredients:	Wt.	C	P	F
4 cups raw cabbage, shredded	400g	40	8	—
1/2 cup celery, chopped	64g	—	—	—
1 small carrot, grated	44g	5	1	—
1 small scallion, minced	20g	—	—	—
1/2 cup dairy sour cream	120g	—	—	20
2 tbsp. tarragon vinegar	30g	—	—	—
1 tbsp. sugar	15g	15	2	—
1/2 tsp. salt	2.5g	—	—	—

Preparation: Combine cabbage, celery, carrot and scallion; refrigerate. Mix rest of ingredients and refrigerate. Just before serving, mix dressing with salad and toss lightly.

Calories: 464 or 58 calories/serving

Servings: 8

Exchange Value: 1/2 bread exchange +
1/2 fat exchange

Nature Salad

Ingredients:	Wt.	C	P	F
3 cups raw cabbage, shredded	300g	30	6	—
1/2 medium cucumber, thinly sliced	50g	5	1	—
1 small onion, thinly sliced	35g	5	1	—
1/2 cup dairy sour cream	120g	—	—	20
2 tbsp. fresh lemon juice	25g	2.5	—	—
1 tsp. sugar	5g	5	.6	—
1 tsp. salt	5g	—	—	—
dash pepper	—	—	—	—

Preparation: Combine all ingredients and toss. Refrigerate.

Calories: 404 or 101 calories/serving
Servings: 4
Exchange Value:

1/2 bread exchange +
1 5% vegetable exchange +
1 fat exchange
            or
1/2 bread exchange +
1/2 fat exchange +
1/4 whole milk exchange (2 ounces)

Main-Dish Fish Salads

Beautiful Days Salad

Ingredients:	Wt.	C	P	F
5 stuffed green olives, chopped	45g	–	–	5
1/2 cup raw carrot, grated	38g	5	.5	–
1/2 cup celery, chopped	64g	–	–	–
1 small onion, minced	35g	5	1	–
1 tbsp. vinegar	15g	–	–	–
1 cup creamed cottage cheese	240g	–	28	20
1/4 tsp. Worcestershire sauce	–	–	–	–
3/4 cup canned tuna, drained and flaked	120g	–	21	15
salt and pepper to taste	–	–	–	–

Preparation: Combine the first 5 ingredients, then mix cottage cheese with Worcestershire sauce. Finally, mix all ingredients together well; season to taste and serve on lettuce.

Calories: 602 or 151 calories/serving
Servings: 4
Exchange Value: 1 1/2 meat exchanges +
1/4 whole milk exchange (2 ounces)
or
2 meat exchanges

Marinated Shrimps

Ingredients:	Wt.	C	P	F
1/4 cup dairy sour cream	60g	–	–	10
1/4 cup chili sauce	60g	17	2	–
2 tsp. horseradish	10g	–	–	–
1/4 tsp. salt	–	–	–	–
30 medium fresh shrimps, cooked, peeled, cleaned and chopped	180g	–	42	30
1 cup celery, chopped	128g	2.5	.5	–

Preparation: Mix together the first 4 ingredients; add shrimps and celery. Serve cold.

Calories: 616 or 154 calories/serving
Servings: 4
Exchange Value: 1 1/2 meat exchanges +
1 5% vegetable exchange +
1/2 fat exchange

Mediterranean Salmon

Ingredients:	Wt.	C	P	F
1 envelope unflavored gelatin	8g	–	–	–
1 cup cold water	200g	–	–	–
1 tbsp. lemon juice	12g	–	–	–
non-caloric liquid sweetener to equal 2 tbsp. sugar	–	–	–	–
1 tbsp. vinegar	15g	–	–	–
1/2 tsp. onion salt	2.5g	–	–	–
1/2 tsp. salt	2.5g	–	–	–
1/4 tsp. horseradish	–	–	–	–
2 cups canned salmon, drained and flaked	320g	–	56	40
3 tbsp. dietetic mayonnaise	45g	–	–	5
3 ounces or 6 tbsp. dairy sour cream	90g	–	–	15
1/2 cup celery, chopped	64g	–	–	–

Preparation: In a medium casserole soften gelatin in cold water. Heat over low heat, stirring constantly, until gelatin is dissolved. Add lemon juice, non-caloric sweetener, vinegar, onion salt, salt and horseradish. Refrigerate until partially set. Fold in rest of ingredients; pour into a 3 1/2-cup mold. Refrigerate until set.

Calories: 764 or 191 calories/serving
Servings: 4
Exchange Value: 2 meat exchanges +
1 fat exchange

Neptune

Ingredients:	Wt.	C	P	F
1 1/2 cups canned tuna, drained and flaked	240g	–	42	30
1 cup clams (canned), drained	240g	–	28	20
2 cups celery, chopped	250g	5	1	–
2 scallions, minced	35g	5	1	–
3 tbsp. pimiento, chopped	45g	5	1	–
3 ounces or 6 tbsp. dietetic mayonnaise	90g	–	–	10
1/2 cup dairy sour cream	120g	–	–	20
1 tbsp. lemon juice	12g	–	–	–
salt and pepper to taste	–	–	–	–

Preparation: Combine the first 5 ingredients; toss lightly. Mix together mayonnaise, sour cream and lemon juice; beat until smooth. Pour over salad and mix well. Season to taste.

Calories: 1072 or 134 calories/serving
Servings: 8
Exchange Value: 1 1/2 meat exchanges + 1/2 fat exchange

Orange Lobster

Ingredients:	Wt.	C	P	F
³/₄ cup canned lobster, drained	120g	–	21	15
2 cups orange quarters	400g	40	4	–
¹/₄ tsp. orange peel, grated	–	–	–	–
2 tbsp. unsweetened orange juice	25g	2.5	–	–
¹/₄ tsp. horseradish	–	–	–	–
¹/₂ envelope dietetic topping for desserts, "Dream Whip," prepared (1 cup)	–	19.2	3.2	–

Preparation: Flake lobster in ¹/₂" (1.25 cm) pieces; sprinkle with salt. Toss with orange sections and refrigerate. Mix grated orange peel, orange juice and horseradish; slowly, fold in dietetic topping. Toss salad lightly with dressing and serve on lettuce bed.

Calories: 495 or 165 calories/serving
Servings: 3
Exchange Value:

1 meat exchange +
1 bread exchange +
1 5% vegetable exchange

Sideboard Salad

Ingredients:	Wt.	C	P	F
6 cups green leaves, torn	420g	30	6	–
1 1/2 cups canned tuna, drained and flaked	240g	–	42	30
1 cup Cheddar cheese, grated (4 ounces)	120g	–	28	20
6 bacon slices, cooked, crisp, drained and crumbled	60g	–	14	10
1/2 cup celery, chopped	64g	–	–	–

Preparation: In a large salad bowl, combine green leaves, tuna, cheese, bacon and celery; toss lightly. Serve with "Onion dressing."*

Calories: 1020 or 255 calories/serving

Servings: 4

Exchange Value: 3 meat exchanges + 1/2 bread exchange

*See Index

Main-Dish Meat-Cheese Salads

American Cottage Cheese

Ingredients:	Wt.	C	P	F
6 cups lettuce leaves, torn	420g	30	6	–
1 cup creamed cottage cheese	240g	–	28	20
2 dill pickles, chopped	100g	–	–	–
1/2 small scallion, minced	10g	–	–	–
2 tsp. salad oil	10g	–	–	10
1 tbsp. vinegar	15g	–	–	–

Preparation: In a large salad bowl, season lettuce to taste. Add cheese, pickles, and scallion. Toss with salad oil and vinegar.

Calories: 526 or 132 calories/serving

Servings: 4

Exchange Value:
1 meat exchange +
1/2 bread exchange +
1/2 fat exchange

Chicken Salad

Ingredients:	Wt.	C	P	F
1½ cups cooked chicken, diced	180g	–	42	30
1 medium cucumber, peeled, halved, seeded and diced	100g	10	2	–
½ cup creamed cottage cheese	120g	–	14	10
½ cup buttermilk	120g	6	4	–
1 tsp. prepared mustard	5g	–	–	–
1 scallion, minced	20g	–	–	–
¾ tsp. salt	3.75g	–	–	–

Preparation: Combine chicken and cucumber. Beat together rest of ingredients and pour dressing over chicken mixture. Toss and refrigerate.

Calories: 672 or 168 calories/serving
Servings: 4
Exchange Value: 2 meat exchanges +
1 5% vegetable exchange

Chief Salad

Ingredients:	Wt.	C	P	F
4 medium cooked potatoes, peeled and cubed	600g	120	16	–
1/2 tsp. salt	2.5g	–	–	–
1/2 cup celery, chopped	64g	–	–	–
1 medium onion, minced	70g	10	1	–
1/2 cup caraway sauce*	120g	12	11.5	12.5
3 ounces or 6 tbsp. dietetic mayonnaise	90g	–	–	10
2 dill pickles, chopped	100g	–	–	–
3 cups lettuce, shredded	210g	15	3	–
4 bologna slices, cut in thin sticks	180g	–	28	20
2 ounces Cheddar cheese, cut in thin sticks	60g	–	14	10
2 ounces Swiss cheese, cut in thin sticks	60g	–	14	10

Preparation: Sprinkle potatoes with salt. Combine potatoes, celery and onion. Mix together caraway sauce, mayonnaise and pickles. Pour half of this dressing over potato mixture; toss lightly, cover and refrigerate. Put lettuce in the bottom of a large salad bowl; arrange potato salad in the centre. Scatter bologna slices and cheeses over contents of bowl. Cover with rest of the sauce.

*Caraway sauce: Gradually, stir 1 tbsp. vinegar into 1/2 cup evaporated milk. Add 2 tbsp. grated Parmesan cheese, 1/4 tsp. salt and 1/4 tsp. caraway seeds. Yielding: 1/2 cup.

Calories: 1541 or 193 calories/serving
Servings: 8
Exchange Value:

	or
1 meat exchange +	1/2 meat exchange +
1 bread exchange +	1 bread exchange +
1 5% vegetable exchange +	1/2 whole milk exchange
1/2 fat exchange	(4 ounces)

Diplomatic Salad

Ingredients:	Wt.	C	P	F
6 cups lettuce leaves, torn	420g	30	6	–
1 medium cucumber, unpeeled, diced	100g	10	2	–
4 ounces cooked ham, cut in strips (1 cup)	120g	–	28	20
4 ounces cooked chicken, cut in strips (1 cup)	120g	–	28	20
2 hard-cooked eggs, sliced	100g	–	14	10
2 medium tomatoes, quartered	180g	10	2	–
3 ounces or 6 tbsp. dietetic mayonnaise	90g	–	–	10
2 tbsp. vinegar	30g	–	–	–
2 tsp. horseradish	10g	–	–	–
1/2 tsp. Worcestershire sauce	2.5g	–	–	–
1/2 tsp. salt	2.5g	–	–	–
dash pepper	–	–	–	–

Preparation: Line small individual bowls with lettuce; equally divide cucumber, ham, chicken, eggs and tomatoes and arrange on top of lettuce. Mix rest of ingredients well and pour them over each salad bowl (1 full tbsp./serving).

Calories: 1060 or 133 calories/serving

Servings: 8

Exchange Value:
1 1/2 meat exchanges +
1 5% vegetable exchange
           or
1 meat exchange +
1/2 fat exchange +
1/2 skimmed milk exchange (4 ounces)

"Hot Buffet" Salad

Ingredients:	Wt.	C	P	F
1 tbsp. butter or margarine	15g	–	–	15
1 tbsp. all-purpose flour	7g	6	.8	–
1 tbsp. sugar	15g	15	2	–
1/2 tsp. garlic salt	2.5g	–	–	–
1/2 tsp. prepared mustard	2.5g	–	–	–
dash pepper	–	–	–	–
1/2 cup water	100g	–	–	–
1/4 cup vinegar	60g	–	–	–
2 cups (8 ounces) cooked ham, cut in fine strips	240g	–	56	40
2 hard-cooked eggs, sliced	100g	–	14	10
1/2 cup celery, chopped	64g	–	–	–
3 cups lettuce leaves, torn	210g	15	3	–
1/2 medium cucumber, unpeeled, thinly sliced	50g	5	1	–
4 ounces (1 cup) Cheddar cheese, cut in thin sticks	120g	–	28	20

Preparation: In a medium skillet, mix the first 6 ingredients well; add water and vinegar and cook over medium heat until boiling point, stirring constantly. To this sauce, add in order: ham, eggs, celery, lettuce, cucumber and cheese. Cover and cook over medium heat 4 to 5 minutes. Remove from heat and toss lightly. Serve immediately.

Calories: 1348 or 225 calories/serving

Servings: 6

Exchange Value:

2 meat exchanges +
1/2 whole milk exchange (4 ounces)

or

2 meat exchanges +
1/2 bread exchange +
1 fat exchange

Pacific Islands Mixture

Ingredients:	Wt.	C	P	F
1 cup canned pineapple pieces, run under water and well drained	250g	20	2	–
4 cups lettuce leaves, torn	280g	20	4	–
4 ounces (1 cup) cooked ham, cubed	120g	–	28	20
14 medium green grapes, fresh, without seeds and halved	70g	10	1	–
2 ounces Swiss cheese (1/2 cup) cut in thin strips	60g	–	14	10
3 ounces unsweetened pineapple juice	80g	10	1	–
3/4 cup dairy sour cream	180g	–	–	30
lettuce	–	–	–	–

Preparation: Combine the first 5 ingredients. Line the bottom of a salad bowl with lettuce and arrange the combined mixture in the centre. Refrigerate. Meanwhile, mix sour cream with pineapple juice and refrigerate. When ready to serve, pour dressing over salad and toss lightly.

Calories: 980 or 163 calories/serving
Servings: 6
Exchange Value:

1 meat exchange +
1 10% vegetable exchange +
1 fat exchange
　　　　or
1 whole milk exchange (8 ounces)
　　　　or
1/2 meat exchange +
1 5% vegetable exchange +
1/2 fat exchange +
1/2 whole milk exchange (4 ounces)

Party Salad

Ingredients:	Wt.	C	P	F
2 medium cooked potatoes, diced	300g	60	8	—
2 hard-cooked eggs, chopped	100g	—	14	10
1 cup celery, chopped	128g	2.5	.5	—
4 1/8" bologna slices (.3125 cm)	180g	—	28	20
1/2 cup Cheddar cheese, diced (2 ounces)	60g	—	14	10
1 cup raw cabbage, shredded	100g	10	2	—
1 scallion, minced	20g	—	—	—
3 ounces or 6 tbsp. dietetic mayonnaise	90g	—	—	10
salt and pepper to taste	—	—	—	—

Preparation: Combine all ingredients except mayonnaise; toss lightly, but thoroughly. Add mayonnaise and toss again. Refrigerate. Serve on green leaves.

Calories: 1006 or 252 calories/serving

Servings: 4

Exchange Value:

2 meat exchanges +
1/2 bread exchange +
1 10% vegetable exchange +
1/2 fat exchange
            or
1 1/2 meat exchanges +
1/2 bread exchange +
1 5% vegetable exchange +
1/2 whole milk exchange (4 ounces)

Stuffed Melons

Ingredients:	Wt.	C	P	F
3 cups cooked chicken, diced	360g	–	84	60
1/2 cup celery, chopped	64g	–	–	–
2 scallions, minced	35g	5	1	–
3/4 tsp. salt	3.75g	–	–	–
1/8 tsp. pepper	–	–	–	–
2 tsp. lemon juice	8g	–	–	–
1/2 tsp. ground ginger	2.5g	–	–	–
6 tbsp. pimiento, chopped	90g	10	2	–
21 fresh green grapes, halved	105g	15	1.5	–
1/2 cup dairy sour cream	120g	–	–	20
2 cantaloups (whole) 5" (12.5 cm) diam.	900g	40	4	–

Preparation: Mix all ingredients together, except cantaloups; cover and refrigerate. When ready to serve, cut cantaloups in half and remove seeds. Cut a very thin slice at the bottom of each melon-half to prevent cantaloup from rolling around the plate. Stuff melons with chicken salad.

Calories: 1370 or 343 calories/serving

Servings: 4

Exchange Value:
3 meat exchanges +
1/2 bread exchange +
1 fruit exchange +
1 fat exchange
      or
2 meat exchanges +
1/2 fruit exchange +
1 whole milk exchange (8 ounces)

Tamed Mushrooms

Ingredients:	Wt.	C	P	F
4 cups cooked beef, cut in strips	480g	–	112	80
6 medium fresh mushrooms, chopped	120g	5	1	–
2 scallions, minced	35g	5	1	–
3 ounces or 6 tbsp. dietetic mayonnaise	90g	–	–	10
1/2 cup dairy sour cream	120g	–	–	20
1/2 tsp. salt	2.5g	–	–	–

Preparation: Combine beef, mushrooms and scallions. Mix mayonnaise, sour cream and salt; toss with meat mixture. Refrigerate. Serve on lettuce leaves.

Calories: 1486 or 248 calories/serving
Servings: 6
Exchange Value: 3 meat exchanges +
1/2 fat exchange

Terrace Delights

Ingredients:	Wt.	C	P	F
1/4 cup chicken broth	56g	–	–	–
2 tsp. curry powder	10g	–	–	–
3 ounces or 6 tbsp. dietetic mayonnaise	90g	–	–	10
1 tbsp. lemon juice	12g	–	–	–
2 1/2 cups cooked chicken, cut in 1" (2.5 cm) strips	300g	–	70	50
1 1/2 cups tangerine quarters	300g	20	2	–
1 cup canned green peas, drained	180g	40	4	–
1/2 cup celery, chopped	64g	–	–	–
1 medium green pepper, chopped	60g	5	1	–
2 scallions, minced	35g	5	1	–

Preparation: In a medium casserole, heat chicken broth; add curry powder and let simmer for 2 minutes. Cool. Add mayonnaise and lemon juice; mix well. Fold in chicken pieces and spoon into the centre of a serving dish; refrigerate. Just before serving, arrange fruits and vegetables around chicken salad.

Calories: 1132 or 189 calories/serving

Servings: 6

Exchange Value:

2 meat exchanges +
1 10% vegetable exchange
        or
1 meat exchange +
1 5% vegetable exchange +
1/2 whole milk exchange (4 ounces)

Tropical Chicken

Ingredients:	Wt.	C	P	F
1 package (3 ounces) pineapple flavored gelatin	85g	90	12	–
1 tsp. garlic salt	5g	–	–	–
1 cup boiling water	200g	–	–	–
1 tsp. onion, grated	5g	–	–	–
1 tbsp. wine vinegar	15g	–	–	–
1/2 cup dairy sour cream	120g	–	–	20
3 ounces or 6 tbsp. dietetic mayonnaise	90g	–	–	10
1 1/2 cups cooked chicken, diced	180g	–	42	30
1/2 cup celery, chopped	64g	–	–	–

Preparation: Dissolve gelatin and garlic salt in boiling water; add onion and vinegar. Let cool. Add sour cream and mayonnaise; mix well. Refrigerate until partially set. Fold in chicken and celery. Pour into a 8"×8"×2" (20 cm×20 cm×5 cm) mold. Refrigerate until set. Cut in squares and serve on lettuce or other green leaves.

Calories: 1116 or 186 calories/serving

Servings: 6

Exchange Value:

1 meat exchange +
1 bread exchange +
1 fat exchange
      or
1/2 meat exchange +
1 10% vegetable exchange +
1/2 fat exchange +
1/2 whole milk exchange (4 ounces)

Main-Dish Fish Molded Salads

Charming Lobster

Ingredients:	Wt.	C	P	F
1 envelope unflavored gelatin	8g	–	–	–
3/4 cup cold water	150g	–	–	–
3/4 cup dairy sour cream	180g	–	–	30
2 tbsp. tarragon vinegar	30g	–	–	–
1/2 tsp. onion salt	2.5g	–	–	–
dash salt	–	–	–	–
1/2 cup canned lobster meat, drained and flaked	80g	–	14	10
1 cup creamed cottage cheese	240g	–	28	20
1/2 medium cucumber, peeled and diced	50g	5	1	–
1/4 cup celery, chopped	32g	–	–	–

Preparation: In a medium casserole, soften gelatin in cold water; heat over low heat, stirring constantly, until dissolved. Let cool. Add sour cream, vinegar, onion salt and salt; beat with an electric mixer until very smooth. Fold in lobster, cottage cheese, cucumber and celery. Pour into a 4 1/2-cup round mold. Refrigerate until firm.

Calories: 732 or 183 calories/serving
Servings: 4
Exchange Value: 1 1/2 meat exchanges +
1 1/2 fat exchanges

Crab Salad

Ingredients:	Wt.	C	P	F
2 envelopes unflavored gelatin	16g	–	–	–
1¹/₂ cups cold water	300g	–	–	–
³/₄ cup chili sauce	180g	51	6	–
3 ounces or 6 tbsp. dietetic mayonnaise	90g	–	–	10
1 cup dairy sour cream	240g	–	–	40
¹/₂ tsp. salt	2.5g	–	–	–
¹/₄ cup lemon juice	50g	5	.5	–
2 scallions, minced	35g	5	1	–
4 hard-cooked eggs, chopped	200g	–	28	20
1 cup celery, chopped	128g	2.5	.5	–
2¹/₂ cups cooked crab meat	400g	–	70	50

Preparation: Soften gelatin in cold water; heat over low heat, stirring constantly, until dissoved. Stir in chili sauce, mayonnaise, sour cream, salt and lemon juice; mix well. Refrigerate until partially set, stirring occasionally. Fold in rest of ingredients. Pour into an 8-cup mold. Refrigerate until firm.

Calories: 1758 or 220 calories/serving
Servings: 8
Exchange Value: 2 meat exchanges +
¹/₂ bread exchange +
1 fat exchange

Fish Salad

Ingredients:	Wt.	C	P	F
1 tbsp. unflavored gelatin	8g	–	–	–
1/4 cup cold water	50g	–	–	–
1 egg	50g	–	7	5
1 tsp. salt	5g	–	–	–
1 tsp. sugar	5g	5	.6	–
1 tsp. flour	2.4g	2	–	–
1/2 tsp. dry mustard	2.5g	–	–	–
2 cups milk	480g	24	16	20
1/2 cup vinegar	120g	–	–	–
4 1/2 ounces cooked fish (haddock, cod, sole, etc.), flaked	135g	–	21	15

Preparation: Soften gelatin in cold water and stir in hot mayonnaise, prepared as follows: beat egg and add rest of dry, mixed ingredients, then the milk and vinegar; cook over low heat, stirring constantly, to prevent curdling. Then, fold in fish and pour into a mold. Refrigerate until set.

Calories: 662 or 166 calories/serving

Servings: 4

Exchange Value:

1 1/2 meat exchanges +
1/2 bread exchange +
1/2 fat exchange

or

1 meat exchange +
1/2 whole milk exchange (4 ounces)

Lobster in Aspic

Ingredients:	Wt.	C	P	F
1 tbsp. unflavored gelatin	8g	–	–	–
2 tbsp. cold water	25g	–	–	–
9 tbsp. dietetic mayonnaise	135g	–	–	15
1/2 cup celery, chopped	64g	–	–	–
1 1/4 cups cooked lobster, flaked	200g	–	35	25
1 tsp. salt	5g	–	–	–
1 tbsp. lemon juice	12g	–	–	–
1/4 cup chili sauce	60g	17	2	–
1 tsp. horseradish	5g	–	–	–

Preparation: Soften gelatin in cold water for 5 minutes, then dissolve over very hot water. Stir in mayonnaise, then fold in rest of ingredients. Pour into individual molds and refrigerate until set. Serve on lettuce leaves.

Calories: 576 or 144 calories/serving
Servings: 4
Exchange Value:

1 meat exchange +
1 5% vegetable exchange +
1 fat exchange
        or
1 meat exchange +
1/2 fat exchange +
1/4 whole milk exchange (2 ounces)

Majestic Tuna

Ingredients:	Wt.	C	P	F
2 envelopes unflavored gelatin	16g	–	–	–
3/4 cup cold water	150g	–	–	–
2 tbsp. vinegar	30g	–	–	–
1/2 tsp. salt	2.5g	–	–	–
2 cups creamed cottage cheese	480g	–	56	40
1 1/2 cups plain yogurt	360g	24	16	10
1 small scallion, minced	20g	–	–	–
3 tbsp. pimiento, chopped	45g	5	1	–
2 cups canned tuna, drained and flaked	320g	–	56	40

Preparation: In a medium casserole, soften gelatin in cold water. Heat over low heat, stirring constantly, until dissoved. Remove from heat; stir in vinegar, salt, cottage cheese and yogurt. Refrigerate until partially set. Fold in scallion, pimiento and tuna. Pour into 6 individual molds or into a 6-cup mold. Refrigerate until firm.

Calories: 1442 or 240 calories/serving
Servings: 6
Exchange Value: 3 meat exchanges +
1 5% vegetable exchange

Molded Tuna

Ingredients:	Wt.	C	P	F
2 envelopes unflavored gelatin	16g	–	–	–
1/2 cup cold water	100g	–	–	–
1 can (10 1/2 ounces) cream of celery soup, undiluted	300g	22.5	3	15
1/4 cup lemon juice	50g	5	.5	–
1 tbsp. prepared mustard	15g	–	–	–
1 tsp. salt	5g	–	–	–
dash pepper	–	–	–	–
3/4 cup dietetic mayonnaise	180g	–	–	20
2 cups canned tuna, drained and flaked	320g	–	56	40
1 cup celery, chopped	128g	2.5	.5	–
1/2 medium cucumber, peeled and grated	50g	5	1	–

Preparation: Soften gelatin in cold water. Heat soup until boiling point; add gelatin, stirring until dissolved. Stir in lemon juice, mustard, salt and pepper. Let cool. Refrigerate until partially set. Stir in mayonnaise and mix well. Fold in rest of ingredients. Pour into a 8 1/2" × 4 1/2" × 2 1/2" (21.25 cm × 11.25 cm × 6.25 cm) mold. Refrigerate until firm.

Calories: 1059 or 132 calories/serving
Servings: 8
Exchange Value:
1 meat exchange +
1 5% vegetable exchange +
1 fat exchange

Seaboard Salad

Ingredients:	Wt.	C	P	F
1 package (3 ounces) lime flavored gelatin	85g	90	12	—
1 cup boiling water	200g	—	—	—
1/2 cup cold water	100g	—	—	—
1 tbsp. vinegar	15g	—	—	—
3 ounces or 6 tbsp. dietetic mayonnaise	90g	—	—	10
1/4 tsp. salt	—	—	—	—
1 medium raw carrot, grated	88g	10	1	—
1 cup raw cabbage, shredded	100g	10	2	—
1/2 tsp. onion powder	2.5g	—	—	—
1 cup canned tuna, drained and flaked	160g	—	28	20

Preparation: Dissolve gelatin in boiling water. Stir in cold water, vinegar, mayonnaise and salt; beat with an electric mixer until smooth. Refrigerate until mixture has the consistency of an egg white (slightly thicker). Pour mixture into a cold bowl and whip until very fluffy. Fold in vegetables and tuna. Pour into 6 individual molds. Refrigerate until set.

Calories: 882 or 147 calories/serving

Servings: 6

Exchange Value:

1 meat exchange +
1 bread exchange
           or
1/2 bread exchange +
1 5% vegetable exchange +
1/2 whole milk exchange (4 ounces)

Shrimps Aspic

Ingredients:	Wt.	C	P	F
1 envelope unflavored gelatin	8g	—	—	—
1/4 cup cold water	50g	—	—	—
1 cup tomato juice	220g	10	2	—
1 cup clam broth	240g	—	—	—
1 tbsp. lemon juice	12g	—	—	—
1 tsp. salt	5g	—	—	—
1/2 tsp. oregano leaves, crushed	2.5g	—	—	—
1/4 tsp. onion powder	—	—	—	—
2 tsp. onion, grated	10g	—	—	—
1/2 cup celery, chopped	64g	—	—	—
15 medium cooked shrimps, cleaned	90g	—	21	15

Preparation: Soften gelatin in cold water. Heat tomato juice, then add gelatin; stir well until dissolved. Add the next 6 ingredients and refrigerate until mixture begins to thicken. Fold in celery and shrimps. Pour into a 1-quart (1 1/8 litres) mold. Refrigerate until set.

Calories: 267 or 45 calories/serving
Servings: 6
Exchange Value: 1/2 meat exchange

Tuna Treasure

Ingredients:	Wt.	C	P	F
1 envelope unflavored gelatin	8g	–	–	–
1/4 cup cold water	50g	–	–	–
1 can (10 1/2 ounces) tomato soup, undiluted	300g	45	6	7.5
1 package (3 ounces) cream cheese	90g	–	–	30
3 ounces or 6 tbsp. dietetic mayonnaise	90g	–	–	10
1/2 cup celery, chopped	64g	–	–	–
5 stuffed green olives, sliced	45g	–	–	5
1 small scallion, minced	20g	–	–	–
3 tbsp. pimiento, chopped	45g	5	1	–
2 hard-cooked eggs, chopped	100g	–	14	10
2 cups canned tuna, drained and flaked	320g	–	56	40

Preparation: Soften gelatin in cold water. Heat soup until boiling point; stir in gelatin and stir until dissolved. Add cream cheese and beat with an electric mixer until very smooth. Add mayonnaise and mix well; fold in rest of ingredients. Pour into a 5-cup mold. Refrigerate until set.

Calories: 1431 or 179 calories/serving
Servings: 8
Exchange Value:

1 meat exchange +
1/2 bread exchange +
1 1/2 fat exchanges
       or
1 meat exchange +
1/2 fat exchange +
1/2 whole milk exchange (4 ounces)
       or
1 1/2 meat exchanges +
1 5% vegetable exchange +
1 fat exchange

Whipped Tuna Jelly

Ingredients:	Wt.	C	P	F
1½ tbsp. unflavored gelatin	12g	–	–	–
½ cup cold water	100g	–	–	–
¼ cup lemon juice	50g	5	.5	–
3 ounces or 6 tbsp. dietetic mayonnaise	90g	–	–	10
2 cups canned tuna, drained and flaked	320g	–	56	40
½ medium cucumber, peeled and chopped	50g	5	1	–
½ cup celery, chopped	64g	–	–	–
10 stuffed green olives, chopped	90g	–	–	10
½ tsp. onion powder	2.5g	–	–	–
1 tsp. horseradish	5g	–	–	–
¼ tsp. salt	–	–	–	–
¼ tsp. paprika	–	–	–	–
1 envelope dietetic topping for desserts "Dream Whip," prepared (2 cups)	–	38.4	6.4	–

Preparation: In a large casserole, soften gelatin in cold water; add lemon juice and heat over medium heat, stirring constantly, until gelatin is dissolved. Fold in mayonnaise and mix well. Add rest of ingredients except dietetic topping. Mix well again, then fold in topping. Pour into a 8½"×4½"×2½" (21.25 cm×11.25 cm×6.25 cm) dish. Refrigerate until set.

Calories: 989 or 124 calories/serving
Servings: 8
Exchange Value:

1 meat exchange +
1 5% vegetable exchange +
½ fat exchange
            or
½ meat exchange +
½ whole milk exchange (4 ounces)

Main-Dish Meat-Cheese Molded Salads

Beef Tongue Mousse

Ingredients:	Wt.	C	P	F
1 tbsp. unflavored gelatin	8g	—	—	—
1/4 cup cold water	50g	—	—	—
1 1/2 tsp. instant beef broth powder or liquid base	7.5g	—	—	—
1 1/4 cups boiling water	250g	—	—	—
1/2 cup heavy cream (35%), whipped	120g	—	—	40
1 tsp. dry mustard	5g	—	—	—
1 tsp. salt	5g	—	—	—
dash pepper	—	—	—	—
1 small onion, minced	35g	5	1	—
1 tbsp. parsley, snipped	3.5g	—	—	—
2 tbsp. lemon juice	25g	2.5	—	—
2 cups cooked beef tongue, chopped	240g	—	56	40

Preparation: Soften gelatin in cold water; add to boiling water along with instant beef broth, stirring until both gelatin and beef broth are well dissolved. Refrigerate until partially set. Mix whipped cream with rest of ingredients and fold in thickened gelatin. Pour into a 9"×5"×3" (22.5 cm×12.5 cm ×7.5 cm) mold. Refrigerate until firm.

Calories: 978 or 122 calories/serving
Servings: 8
Exchange Value: 1 meat exchange + 1 fat exchange

Chicken and Sour Cream

Ingredients:	Wt.	C	P	F
1 envelope unflavored gelatin	8g	–	–	–
1/4 cup cold water	50g	–	–	–
1 cup hot chicken broth	225g	–	–	–
1 1/2 cups cooked chicken, diced	180g	–	42	30
1/4 cup celery, chopped	32g	–	–	–
56 fresh green grapes, halved	280g	40	4	–
3/4 cup dairy sour cream	180g	–	–	30
1 tbsp. parsley, snipped	3.5g	–	–	–
1/2 scallion, minced	10g	–	–	–
1/2 tsp. thyme leaves, crushed	2.5g	–	–	–

Preparation: Soften gelatin in cold water and dissolve in hot broth. Let cool; add rest of ingredients and mix well. Pour into a 5-cup mold. Refrigerate until set.

Calories: 884 or 147 calories/serving

Servings: 6

Exchange Value:
1 meat exchange +
1/2 bread exchange +
1 fat exchange
            or
1/2 meat exchange +
1/2 fat exchange +
1/2 whole milk exchange (4 ounces)

Fancy Ham Squares

Ingredients:	Wt.	C	P	F
1 1/2 cups cooked ham, diced	180g	—	42	30
1/4 cup chili sauce	60g	17	2	—
1/2 tsp. onion powder	2.5g	—	—	—
2 tsp. prepared mustard	10g	—	—	—
1/2 tsp. horseradish	2.5g	—	—	—
1 envelope unflavored gelatin	8g	—	—	—
1/2 cup cold water	100g	—	—	—
3 ounces or 6 tbsp. dietetic mayonnaise	90g	—	—	10
2 medium cooked potatoes, peeled and diced	300g	60	8	—
1/2 cup celery, chopped	64g	—	—	—
1/2 small scallion, minced	10g	—	—	—
2 tsp. vinegar	10g	—	—	—
1 tsp. salt	5g	—	—	—
dash pepper	—	—	—	—

Preparation: Combine the first 5 ingredients. In a small casserole, soften gelatin in cold water; heat over low heat, stirring constantly, until dissolved. Add mayonnaise and mix well; pour half of gelatin mixture into ham mixture. Pour into a 10" x 6" x 1 1/2" (25 cm x 3.75 cm) dish; refrigerate until almost set. Keep other gelatin half at room temperature. Mix rest of ingredients and add gelatin you kept aside. Pour this over the almost-set ham layer. Refrigerate until firm.

Calories: 876 or 219 calories/serving
Servings: 4
Exchange Value:

	or
1 meat exchange +	1 1/2 meat exchanges +
1/2 bread exchange +	1 bread exchange +
1 5% vegetable exchange +	1 5% vegetable exchange +
1/2 whole milk exchange	1/2 fat exchange
(4 ounces)	

Frothy Ham

Ingredients:	Wt.	C	P	F
2 envelopes unflavored gelatin	16g	–	–	–
1/2 cup cold water	100g	–	–	–
2 medium egg yolks, beaten	34g	–	6	10
1/2 tsp. salt	2.5g	–	–	–
1/4 tsp. onion powder	–	–	–	–
1/2 tsp. dry mustard	2.5g	–	–	–
1 cup milk	240g	12	8	10
1 cup hot water	200g	–	–	–
1 tsp. instant chicken broth powder or liquid base	5g	–	–	–
2 cups cooked ham, ground	240g	–	56	40
1 tsp. paprika	5g	–	–	–
1 tsp. cider vinegar	5g	–	–	–
1 tbsp. parsley, snipped	3.5g	–	–	–
1/2 envelope dietetic topping for desserts "Dream Whip," prepared (1 cup)	–	19.2	3.2	–

Preparation: Soften gelatin in cold water; combine the next 7 ingredients in a double-boiler. Cook over very hot water (but not boiling), stirring constantly, for 15 minutes or until mixture coats a metal spoon. Stir in gelatin, ham, paprika, vinegar and parsley. Refrigerate until moderately set. Fold in topping and pour into a 6-cup mold. Refrigerate until firm.

Calories: 958 or 120 calories/serving
Servings: 8
Exchange Value:

1 meat exchange + 1/4 whole milk exchange (2 ounces)	or 1 meat exchange + 1 5% vegetable exchange + 1/2 fat exchange

Gourmet Salad

Ingredients:	Wt.	C	P	F
1 envelope unflavored gelatin	8g	–	–	–
1 cup cold water, divided equally into two containers	200g	–	–	–
1 can (10½ ounces) cream of mushroom soup, undiluted	300g	22.5	3	30
1 tbsp. lemon juice	12g	–	–	–
dash pepper	–	–	–	–
½ cup cooked chicken, diced	60g	–	14	10
½ cup celery, chopped	64g	–	–	–
2 tbsp. pimiento, chopped	30g	–	–	–
1 small scallion, minced	20g	–	–	–

Preparation: Soften gelatin in ½ cup cold water. Heat over low heat, stirring constantly, until dissolved. Remove from heat; add soup and mix well until very smooth. Stir in the other ½ cup cold water, lemon juice and pepper. Refrigerate until partially set. Fold in rest of ingredients. Pour into a 3-cup mold and refrigerate until firm.

Calories: 518 or 130 calories/serving
Servings: 4
Exchange Value:

½ meat exchange +
1 5% vegetable exchange +
1½ fat exchanges
      or
1 fat exchange +
½ whole milk exchange (4 ounces)

Ham-Cabbage Marinated Jelly

Ingredients:	Wt.	C	P	F
1 package (3 ounces) lemon flavored gelatin	85g	90	12	—
1/2 tsp. salt	2.5g	—	—	—
1 cup boiling water	200g	—	—	—
1/2 cup cold water	100g	—	—	—
1 tbsp. vinegar	15g	—¿	—	—
3 tbsp. dietetic mayonnaise	45g	—	—	5
1 tsp. prepared mustard	5g	—	—	—
1 1/2 cups cooked ham, diced	180g	—	42	30
1 cup raw cabbage, shredded	100g	10	2	—
1 small scallion, minced	20g	—	—	—

Preparation: Dissolve gelatin and salt in boiling water; stir in cold water and vinegar. Let cool, then fold in mayonnaise and mustard and mix well. Refrigerate until partially set. Fold in ham, cabbage and scallion. Pour into 6 individual molds. Refrigerate until firm.

Calories: 939 or 157 calories/serving

Servings: 6

Exchange Value:

1 meat exchange +
1/2 bread exchange +
1 10% vegetable exchange
            or
1 5% vegetable exchange +
1 fat exchange +
1 skimmed milk exchange (8 ounces)

Harmonious Molded Mixture

Ingredients:	Wt.	C	P	F
1½ tbsp. unflavored gelatin	12g	–	–	–
2 cups cold water	400g	–	–	–
½ tsp. salt	2.5g	–	–	–
dash pepper	–	–	–	–
dash paprika	–	–	–	–
1½ cups cooked chicken, cubed	180g	–	42	30
1 cup cooked rice	210g	45	6	–
½ cup celery, chopped	64g	–	–	–
½ medium dill pickle, chopped	25g	–	–	–
10 stuffed green olives, thinly sliced	90g	–	–	10
1 tbsp. parsley, snipped	3.5g	–	–	–
3 ounces or 6 tbsp. dietetic mayonnaise	90g	–	–	10
½ cup heavy cream (35%), whipped	120g	–	–	40

Preparation: In a medium casserole, soften gelatin in cold water; heat over low heat, stirring constantly, until dissolved. Add salt, pepper and paprika. Mix in chicken well with rest of ingredients, then fold in dissolved gelatin. Pour into a 8"×8"×2" (20 cm ×20cm×5 cm) mold. Refrigerate until set.

Calories: 1182 or 197 calories/serving
Servings: 6
Exchange Value:
1 meat exchange +
½ bread exchange +
2 fat exchanges

Lovers' Salad

Ingredients:	Wt.	C	P	F
1¼ cups creamed cottage cheese	300g	–	35	25
1 package (6 ounces) cream cheese, softened	180g	–	–	60
1 tsp. unflavored gelatin	2.6g	–	–	–
¼ cup cold water	50g	–	–	–
¼ tsp. salt	–	–	–	–
28 fresh green grapes, without seeds	140g	20	2	–
1 small scallion, minced	20g	–	–	–
1 envelope dietetic topping for desserts "Dream Whip," prepared (2 cups)	–	38.4	6.4	–

Preparation: Mash together cottage cheese and cream cheese. Soften gelatin in cold water; dissolve over very hot water, then add salt. Add gelatin mixture to cheese mixture. Fold in grapes and scallion, then topping. Pour into a 5-cup, crown-form mold. Refrigerate until set.

Calories: 1172 or 147 calories/serving

Servings: 8

Exchange Value:
1 meat exchange +
½ bread exchange +
1 fat exchange
           or
½ meat exchange +
½ fat exchange +
½ whole milk exchange (4 ounces)

Molded Chicken Surprise

Ingredients:	Wt.	C	P	F
1 envelope unflavored gelatin	8g	—	—	—
1 1/2 cups unsweetened pineapple juice	320g	40	4	—
1/2 tsp. salt	2.5g	—	—	—
3/4 cup plain yogurt	180g	12	8	5
3 tbsp. dietetic mayonnaise	45g	—	—	5
1 1/2 cups cooked chicken, diced	180g	—	42	30
1/2 cup celery, chopped	64g	—	—	—

Preparation: In a small casserole, soften gelatin in pineapple juice; add salt. Heat over low heat, stirring constantly, until dissolved. Mix yogurt with mayonnaise; stir in gelatin mixture. Refrigerate until partially set. Fold in chicken and celery. Pour into 4 individual molds and refrigerate until firm.

Calories: 784 or 196 calories/serving
Servings: 4
Exchange Value:

2 meat exchanges +
1/2 bread exchange +
1 5% vegetable exchange
or
1 meat exchange +
1/2 bread exchange +
1/2 whole milk exchange (4 ounces)

Salad Loaf

Ingredients:	Wt.	C	P	F
1/4 cup cold water	50g	–	–	–
1/2 cup tomato juice	110g	5	.5	–
1 envelope unflavored gelatin	8g	–	–	–
3/4 lb. cooked chicken livers	360g	–	84	60
1 cup tomato juice	220g	10	1	–
3 ounces or 6 tbsp. dietetic mayonnaise	90g	–	–	10
2 tbsp. lemon juice	25g	2.5	–	–
2 tsp. sugar	10g	10	1.2	–
1/2 tsp. salt	2.5g	–	–	–
1/2 tsp. dry mustard	2.5g	–	–	–
1/8 tsp. pepper	–	–	–	–
1/8 tsp. ground cloves	–	–	–	–
1/2 cup celery, chopped	64g	–	–	–
10 stuffed green olives, chopped	90g	–	–	10
2 scallions, minced	35g	5	1	–

Preparation: Mix water with 1/2 cup tomato juice; sprinkle with gelatin to soften. Heat over low heat, stirring constantly, until dissolved. Refrigerate until partially set. Mash chicken livers thoroughly with back of fork and add to gelatin, along with rest of ingredients. Mix everything together well to obtain as smooth a mixture as possible. Pour into a 9″×5″×3″ (22.5 cm×12.5 cm×7.5 cm) mold. Refrigerate until firm.

Calories: 1201 or 200 calories/serving
Servings: 6
Exchange Value:

	or
2 meat exchanges + 1 5% vegetable exchange + 1/2 fat exchange	1 1/2 meat exchanges + 1/2 whole milk exchange (4 ounces)

Soft Creamed Cottage Cheese

Ingredients:	Wt.	C	P	F
1 envelope unflavored gelatin	8g	–	–	–
1 tbsp. sugar	15g	15	2	–
1/2 tsp. salt	2.5g	–	–	–
1/2 cup water	100g	–	–	–
1 1/2 cups creamed cottage cheese	360g	–	42	30
1/2 envelope dietetic topping for desserts "Dream Whip," prepared (1 cup)	–	19.2	3.2	–
4 raw small pears, unpeeled, diced	300g	40	4	–

Preparation: Combine gelatin, sugar, salt and water in a double boiler. Heat over boiling water, stirring constantly, until gelatin is dissolved. Add rest of ingredients. Pour into a 1-quart (1 1/8 litre) mold. Refrigerate until firm.

Calories: 772 or 129 calories/serving
Servings: 6
Exchange Value: 1 meat exchange +
1/2 bread exchange +
1 5% vegetable exchange

Velvety Chicken Salad

Ingredients:	Wt.	C	P	F
2 envelopes unflavored gelatin	16g	–	–	–
2¼ cups chicken broth	506g	–	–	–
2 tbsp. Worcestershire sauce	30g	–	–	–
1 tbsp. lemon juice	12g	–	–	–
dash salt	–	–	–	–
dash paprika	–	–	–	–
2½ cups cooked chicken, diced	300g	–	70	50
½ cup celery, chopped	64g	–	–	–
1½ cups dairy sour cream	360g	–	–	60

Preparation: Soften gelatin in 1 cup chicken broth; heat over medium heat until dissolved. Add rest of chicken broth, Worcestershire sauce, lemon juice, salt and paprika. Refrigerate until partially set. Fold in rest of ingredients. Pour into a 1½ quart (1⅝ litre) mold. Refrigerate until firm.

Calories: 1270 or 127 calories/serving
Servings: 10
Exchange Value: 1 meat exchange +
1 fat exchange

Potato Salads

Artistic Potatoes

Ingredients:	Wt.	C	P	F
1 envelope unflavored gelatin	8g	–	–	–
2 tbsp. sugar	30g	30	4	–
1 tsp. salt	5g	–	–	–
1 1/4 cups boiling water	250g	–	–	–
1/4 cup lemon juice	50g	5	.5	–
5 stuffed green olives, sliced	45g	–	–	5
3 hard-cooked eggs, chopped	150g	–	21	15
4 medium cooked potatoes, peeled and diced	600g	120	16	–
1/2 cup celery, chopped	64g	–	–	–
3 tbsp. pimiento, chopped	45g	5	1	–
1 small scallion, minced	20g	–	–	–
2 tbsp. parsley, snipped	7g	–	–	–
1 1/2 tsp. salt	7.5g	–	–	–
3/4 cup dietetic mayonnaise	180g	–	–	20
1/2 envelope dietetic topping for desserts "Dream Whip," prepared (1 cup)	–	19.2	3.2	–

Preparation: Mix gelatin, sugar and salt well; pour boiling water over this mixture and stir until gelatin and sugar are well dissolved. Add lemon juice; refrigerate until partially set. Fold in rest of ingredients and pour into a 6-cup, crown-form mold. Refrigerate until firm.

Calories: 1260 or 158 calories/serving
Servings: 8
Exchange Value:

1/2 meat exchange + 1 1/2 bread exchanges + 1/2 fat exchange	or 1 bread exchange + 1/2 whole milk exchange (4 ounces)

Eccentric Potato Salad

Ingredients:	Wt.	C	P	F
2 tbsp. vinegar	30g	—	—	—
1/2 tsp. celery seeds	2.5g	—	—	—
1/2 tsp. mustard seeds	2.5g	—	—	—
3 medium potatoes	450g	90	12	—
2 tsp. sugar	10g	10	1.3	—
1/2 tsp. salt	2.5g	—	—	—
2 cups raw cabbage, shredded	200g	20	4	—
1 1/2 cups canned pressed meat (luncheon meat), cubed	270g	—	42	30
2 scallions, sliced	35g	5	1	—
2 medium dill pickles, chopped	100g	—	—	—
3 ounces or 6 tbsp. dietetic mayonnaise	90g	—	—	10
1/4 cup whole milk	60g	3	2	2.5

Preparation: Mix vinegar, celery and mustard seeds; set aside. Meanwhile, peel and cook potatoes in boiling, salted water; drain, then cube. Drizzle potatoes with vinegar mixture; sprinkle with sugar and salt, and refrigerate. Just before serving, add meat, scallions and pickles. Mix mayonnaise, milk and 1/2 tsp. salt; pour this dressing over salad and toss lightly.

Calories: 1144 or 191 calories/serving

Servings: 6

Exchange Value:
1 meat exchange +
1 1/2 bread exchanges +
1/2 fat exchange
            or
1/2 meat exchange +
1 bread exchange +
1/2 whole milk exchange (4 ounces)

"Hostess" Potatoes

Ingredients:	Wt.	C	P	F
non-caloric sweetener to equal 1/3 cup sugar	–	–	–	–
1 tbsp. cornstarch	8g	7.5	1	–
1/2 cup milk	120g	6	4	5
1/4 cup vinegar	60g	–	–	–
1 egg	50g	–	7	5
1 tbsp. butter or margarine	15g	–	–	15
1/2 tsp. celery seeds	2.5g	–	–	–
1/4 tsp. dry mustard	–	–	–	–
3/4 tsp. salt	3.75g	–	–	–
1 small onion, minced	35g	5	1	–
3 tbsp. dietetic mayonnnaise	45g	–	–	5
6 medium cooked potatoes, peeled and diced	900g	180	24	–
3 hard-cooked eggs, chopped	150g	–	21	15

Preparation: In a medium casserole, combine the first 9 ingredients. Cook over low heat, stirring until bubbling. Remove from heat; add onion and mayonnaise. Let cool. Mix potatoes with eggs and fold gently into sauce. Refrigerate.

Calories: 1431 or 239 calories/serving
Servings: 6
Exchange Value:

1 meat exchange +
2 bread exchanges +
1/2 fat exchange
        or
1/2 meat exchange +
1 bread exchange +
1 10% vegetable exchange +
1/2 whole milk exchange (4 ounces)

Novelty Potatoes

Ingredients:	Wt.	C	P	F
5 medium cooked potatoes, peeled and cubed	750g	150	20	–
1 cup celery, finely chopped	128g	2.5	–	–
4 hard-cooked eggs, chopped	200g	–	28	20
1 scallion, minced	20g	–	–	–
1 cup dairy sour cream	240g	–	–	40
1/4 cup evaporated milk	60g	6	4	5
1/4 cup Danish blue cheese, crumbled (1 ounce)	30g	–	7	5
2 tbsp. vinegar	30g	–	–	–
1/4 tsp. dry mustard	–	–	–	–
dash pepper	–	–	–	–

Preparation: Sprinkle potatoes with 1 tsp. salt. Combine potatoes, celery, eggs, and scallion. Mix together rest of ingredients and pour over potato mixture. Toss lightly and refrigerate.

Calories: 1500 or 150 calories/serving
Servings: 10
Exchange Value:

1/2 meat exchange +
1 bread exchange +
1 fat exchange
            or
1 fruit exchange +
1/2 fat exchange +
1/2 whole milk exchange (4 ounces)

Parmentier Salad

Ingredients:	Wt.	C	P	F
3 ounces or 6 tbsp. dietetic mayonnaise	90g	–	–	10
1 tbsp. vinegar	15g	–	–	–
1/2 tsp. Worcestershire sauce	2.5g	–	–	–
1/4 tsp. prepared mustard	–	–	–	–
2 medium cooked potatoes, peeled and diced	300g	60	8	–
2 hard-cooked eggs, chopped	100g	–	14	10
2 cups creamed cottage cheese	480g	–	56	40
3 tbsp. pimiento, chopped	45g	5	1	–
1 small scallion, minced	20g	–	–	–
parsley, snipped, to taste	–	–	–	–
1 tsp. salt	5g	–	–	–

Preparation: Mix mayonnaise, vinegar, Worcestershire sauce and mustard; add potatoes and eggs. Let stand a few minutes. Add rest of ingredients; toss lightly but thoroughly. Pour into a round or a crown-form mold and refrigerate.

Calories: 1116 or 186 calories/serving
Servings: 6
Exchange Value:
2 meat exchanges +
1 10% vegetable exchange
          or
1 1/2 meat exchanges +
1/2 bread exchange +
1/4 whole milk exchange (2 ounces)

Potato Salad

Ingredients:	Wt.	C	P	F
2 tbsp. vinegar	30g	–	–	–
1 1/2 tsp. salt	7.5g	–	–	–
dash pepper	–	–	–	–
4 medium cooked potatoes, peeled, hot and diced	600g	120	16	–
24 medium, ripe olives, chopped	240g	–	–	40
2 hard-cooked eggs, diced	100g	–	14	10
1 cup celery, sliced (thinly)	128g	2.5	.5	–
3 tbsp. pimiento, chopped	45g	5	1	–
1 medium dill pickle, finely chopped	50g	–	–	–
1 small onion, minced	35g	5	1	–
3 ounces or 6 tbsp. dietetic mayonnaise	90g	–	–	10

Preparation: Mix the first 3 ingredients well; pour over potatoes and toss. Let cool before adding olives and rest of ingredients. Toss again and refrigerate.

Calories: 1200 or 200 calories/serving
Servings: 6
Exchange Value:

1/2 meat exchange +
1 1/2 bread exchanges +
1 1/2 fat exchanges
          or
1 bread exchange +
1 fat exchange +
1/2 whole milk exchange (4 ounces)

Potatoes, Hungarian Style

Ingredients:	Wt.	C	P	F
¼ cup dairy sour cream	60g	–	–	10
3 tbsp. dietetic mayonnaise	45g	–	–	5
3 medium cooked potatoes, peeled and diced	450g	90	12	–
1 tsp. scallion, minced	5g	–	–	–
3 bacon slices, cooked, crisp and drained	30g	–	7	5
salt and papper to taste	–	–	–	–

Preparation: Mix sour cream and mayonnaise. Add them to the potatoes; fold in rest of ingredients. Toss lightly but thoroughly. Season to taste and serve on lettuce leaves, if desired.

Calories: 616 or 154 calories/serving
Servings: 4
Exchange Value: 1½ bread exchanges +
1 fat exchange

Potatoes on Stage

Ingredients:	Wt.	C	P	F
12 small cooked potatoes, peeled and cubed	900g	180	24	–
6 medium apples, unpeeled and diced	900g	120	12	–
1 small onion, minced	35g	5	1	–
3/4 cup dairy sour cream	180g	–	–	30
1 1/2 tbsp. lemon juice	18g	–	–	–
1/2 tsp. salt	2.5g	–	–	–
dash pepper	–	–	–	–

Preparation: Combine potatoes, apples, onion and seasonings in a salad bowl. Mix sour cream well with lemon juice and pour over potato mixture. Toss carefully. Refrigerate for a few hours before serving.

Calories: 1638 or 205 calories/serving
Servings: 8
Exchange Value: 2 bread exchanges +
1 fruit exchange +
1/2 fat exchange

Sharp Potato Salad

Ingredients:	Wt.	C	P	F
5 beef sausages (hot dog), sliced ¹/₂" (1.25 cm) thick	180g	–	42	30
2 tsp. butter or margarine	10g	–	–	10
¹/₂ envelope dry onion soup mix	–	15	2	–
1 tbsp. all-purpose flour	7g	6	.8	–
1 tbsp. sugar	15g	15	2	–
¹/₂ cup water	100g	–	–	–
2 tbsp. vinegar	30g	–	–	–
4 medium cooked potatoes, peeled and sliced	600g	120	16	–
¹/₂ cup dairy sour cream	120g	–	–	20

Preparation: In a skillet, cook sausages in melted butter or margarine; remove from heat. Add soup mix, flour, sugar, water and vinegar. Heat again and cook, stirring constantly, until boiling point. Reduce heat, cover and let simmer gently for 10 minutes. Add potatoes and sour cream; heat through and serve.

Calories: 1415 or 236 calories/serving
Servings: 6
Exchange Value:

1 meat exchange +
1 bread exchange +
1 10% vegetable exchange +
1 fat exchange
          or
1 bread exchange +
1 whole milk exchange (8 ounces)

Skillet Potatoes

Ingredients:	Wt.	C	P	F
6 medium cooked potatoes, peeled and diced	900g	180	24	–
6 bacon slices	60g	14	10	–
2 tbsp. bacon fat	30g	–	–	30
1 medium onion, minced	70g	10	1	–
1 can (10 1/2 ounces) cream of celery soup, undiluted	300g	22.5	3	15
1/2 cup milk	120g	6	4	5
1 tbsp. unsweetened relish	15g	–	–	–
2 tbsp. vinegar	30g	–	–	–
1/2 tsp. salt	2.5g	–	–	–
parsley	–	–	–	–

Preparation: Keep potatoes warm. In a large skillet, cook bacon until very crisp; drain all fat but 2 tbsp. Crumble bacon and set aside. Add to bacon fat the minced onion and cook just until tender. Stir in soup, milk, relish, vinegar and salt. Heat until boiling point, stirring constantly. Gently fold in potatoes and crumbled bacon; heat through. Garnish with parsley if desired.

Calories: 1598 or 266 calories/serving
Servings: 6
Exchange Value:

2 bread exchanges +
1 fat exchange +
1/2 whole milk exchange (4 ounces)
      or
1/2 meat exchange +
2 bread exchanges +
1 5% vegetable exchange +
1 1/2 fat exchanges

Specialized Potatoes

Ingredients:	Wt.	C	P	F
12 small, cooked potatoes, peeled and cubed	900g	180	24	—
1/2 medium cucumber, diced	50g	5	1	—
1 small onion, minced	35g	5	1	—
3 tbsp. pimiento, chopped	45g	5	1	—
1 1/2 tsp. salt	7.5g	—	—	—
dash pepper	—	—	—	—
2 hard-cooked eggs, chopped	100g	—	14	10
1/2 envelope dietetic topping for desserts "Dream Whip," prepared (1 cup)	—	19.2	3.2	—
3 ounces or 6 tbsp. dietetic mayonnaise	90g	—	—	10
2 tbsp. vinegar	30g	—	—	—
1 tbsp. prepared mustard	15g	—	—	—

Preparation: Combine the first 7 ingredients. Mix topping with mayonnaise, vinegar and mustard. Add to salad and toss carefully. Refrigerate a few hours before serving on lettuce leaves.

Calories: 1214 or 121 calories/serving

Servings: 10

Exchange Value:
1 1/2 bread exchanges +
1/2 fat exchange
        or
1/2 meat exchange +
2 fruit exchanges

Pasta Salads

Confetti Rice

Ingredients:	Wt.	C	P	F
3 cups cooked rice	630g	135	18	—
5 hard-cooked eggs, finely chopped	250g	—	35	25
1 medium onion, minced	70g	10	1	—
2 tbsp. pimiento, chopped	30g	—	—	—
1/2 cup celery, chopped	64g	—	—	—
dash pepper	—	—	—	—
2 medium dill pickles, finely chopped	100g	—	—	—
1 tsp. salt	5g	—	—	—
3 tbsp. dietetic mayonnaise	45g	—	—	5
1 tsp. vinegar	5g	—	—	—
1 tsp. lemon juice	4g	—	—	—
4 tsp. prepared mustard	20g	—	—	—

Preparation: Combine the first 8 ingredients. Mix mayonnaise, vinegar, lemon juice and mustard well; add to rice mixture and toss. Serve, cooled, in lettuce cups.

Calories: 1066 or 213 calories/serving
Servings: 5
Exchange Value:
1 meat exchange +
2 bread exchanges

Delicious Macaroni and Cheese

Ingredients:	Wt.	C	P	F
4 cups cooked shell macaroni	560g	120	16	–
1 cup creamed cottage cheese	240g	–	28	20
2 tbsp. pimiento, chopped	30g	–	–	–
1 small scallion, minced	20g	–	–	–
1/2 cup dairy sour cream	120g	–	–	20
1 tbsp. lemon juice	12g	–	–	–
1/4 tsp. salt	–	–	–	–
2 ounces Cheddar cheese (1/2 cup), grated	60g	–	14	10

Preparation: Add to the well-drained macaroni, the rest of the ingredients and toss briskly.

Calories: 1162 or 232 calories/serving
Servings: 5
Exchange Value:

1 meat exchange +
1 bread exchange +
1 fruit exchange +
1 fat exchange
    or
1/2 bread exchange +
1 5% vegetable exchange +
1 whole milk exchange (8 ounces)
    or
1 meat exchange +
1 bread exchange +
1/2 whole milk exchange (4 ounces)

Exotic Macaroni

Ingredients:	Wt.	C	P	F
4 cups cooked elbow macaroni	560g	120	16	–
1 cup canned tuna, drained and flaked	160g	–	28	20
2 canned peach halves, run under water, drained and chopped	155g	10	1	–
10 walnuts, finely chopped	14g	–	–	10
3/4 cup dairy sour cream	180g	–	–	30
salt and pepper to taste	–	–	–	–

Preparation: Combine all ingredients. Toss gently but thoroughly. Refrigerate.

Calories: 1240 or 207 calories/serving
Servings: 6
Exchange Value:
1 meat exchange +
1 bread exchange +
1/2 fruit exchange +
1 fat exchange

Gabrielle Macaroni

Ingredients:	Wt.	C	P	F
1 small can (3 ounces) of sliced mushrooms	90g	3.75	.75	–
6 bacon slices	60g	–	14	10
2 tbsp. bacon fat	30g	–	–	30
non-caloric liquid sweetener to equal 1/2 cup sugar	–	–	–	–
2 1/2 tbsp. all-purpose flour	18g	15	2	–
1/4 cup vinegar	60g	–	–	–
1/2 tsp. salt	2.5g	–	–	–
dash pepper	–	–	–	–
1 cup uncooked macaroni	120g	60	8	–
1 small scallion, minced	20g	–	–	–
1/2 cup celery, finely chopped	64g	–	–	–

Preparation: Drain mushrooms and keep liquid; add just enough water to the mushroom liquid to make 1 cup. In a large casserole, fry bacon until very crisp; drain all fat but 2 tbsp. Crumble bacon and set aside. Combine flour, salt and pepper and mix with bacon fat in the casserole. Mix vinegar, non-caloric sweetener and the reserved liquid. Add to flour mixture and cook until sauce thickens and bubbles. Meanwhile, cook macaroni and drain well. In the casserole, lightly toss the macaroni with the sauce, the mushrooms, the crumbled bacon, the minced scallion and the chopped celery. Serve immediately.

Calories: 774 or 97 calories/serving
Servings: 8
Exchange Value:
1/2 meat exchange +
1 10% vegetable exchange +
1/2 fat exchange

Macaroni and Company

Ingredients:	Wt.	C	P	F
4 cups elbow macaroni, cooked	560g	120	16	—
³/₄ cup dairy sour cream	180g	—	—	30
salt and pepper to taste	—	—	—	—
9 bacon slices, crisply cooked, drained and crumbled	90g	—	21	15
1 cup cooked chicken, diced	120g	—	28	20
2 hard-cooked eggs, chopped	100g	—	14	10
3 tbsp. pimiento, chopped	45g	5	1	—
2 tbsp. lemon juice	25g	2.5	—	—

Preparation: Combine all ingredients; toss carefully but thoroughly. Refrigerate.

Calories: 1505 or 251 calories/serving
Servings: 6
Exchange Value:

1 ¹/₂ meat exchanges +
1 ¹/₂ bread exchanges +
1 fat exchange
          or
¹/₂ meat exchange +
1 10% vegetable exchange +
1 whole milk exchange (8 ounces)
          or
1 meat exchange +
1 bread exchange +
¹/₂ fat exchange +
¹/₂ whole milk exchange (4 ounces)

Macaroni of Opportunity

Ingredients:	Wt.	C	P	F
4 cups cooked elbow macaroni	560g	120	16	—
1 cup celery, thinly sliced	128g	2.5	.5	—
1/2 medium cucumber, peeled and diced	50g	5	1	—
2 scallions, minced	35g	5	1	—
2 tbsp. parsley, minced	7g	—	—	—
9 tbsp. dietetic mayonnaise	135g	—	—	15
2 tbsp. vinegar	30g	—	—	—
2 tsp. prepared mustard	10g	—	—	—
1 1/2 tsp. salt	7.5g	—	—	—
dash pepper	—	—	—	—

Preparation: Mix all ingredients well and refrigerate.

Calories: 739 or 123 calories/serving
Servings: 6
**Exchange
Value:** 1 1/2 bread exchanges +
1/2 fat exchange

Macaroni Stuffed Green Peppers

Ingredients:	Wt.	C	P	F
2 cups cooked macaroni	280g	60	8	–
8 medium green peppers	480g	40	8	–
1 1/2 cups cooked ham, cubed	180g	–	42	30
1 cup Cheddar cheese (4 ounces), diced	120g	–	28	20
2 medium dill pickles, diced	100g	–	–	–
2 tbsp. pimiento, chopped	30g	–	–	–
1 small scallion, minced	20g	–	–	–
3 ounces or 6 tbsp. dietetic mayonnaise	90g	–	–	10
2 tsp. prepared mustard	10g	–	–	–
1/4 tsp. salt	–	–	–	–

Preparation: Cut top off green peppers; remove seeds and membrane. Cook peppers in boiling, salted water for 5 minutes, then immerse them immediately in cold water. Mix macaroni, ham, cheese, pickles, pimiento and scallion. Mix together mayonnaise, mustard and salt; pour over macaroni salad and toss lightly. Salt inside of peppers and stuff them with macaroni mixture. Refrigerate and serve on lettuce leaves.

Calories: 1284 or 161 calories/serving

Servings: 8

Exchange Value:

1 meat exchange +
1/2 bread exchange +
1 5% vegetable exchange +
1/2 fat exchange

or

1/2 meat exchange +	1/2 meat exchange +
1/2 bread exchange +	1 fat exchange +
1/2 whole milk exchange	1 skimmed milk exchange
(4 ounces)	(8 ounces)

Rice of Korea

Ingredients:	Wt.	C	P	F
3 cups cooked rice	630g	135	18	—
3 tbsp. dietetic mayonnaise	45g	—	—	5
7 tsp. salad oil	35g	—	—	35
1/4 cup vinegar	60g	—	—	—
1 small onion, grated	35g	5	1	—
3/4 tsp. salt	3.75g	—	—	—
1/8 tsp. pepper	—	—	—	—
2 tsp. horseradish	10g	—	—	—
2 cups cooked beets, diced	300g	40	4	—

Preparation: Throroughly mix mayonnaise with the next 6 ingredients; add rice and beets. Toss and refrigerate for 1 hour. Serve on green leaves.

Calories: 1172 or 147 calories/serving
Servings: 8
Exchange Value:

1 1/2 bread exchanges +
1 fat exchange
          or
1/2 bread exchange +
1 10% vegetable exchange +
1 5% vegetable exchange +
1 fat exchange

Spiced Rice Salad

Ingredients:	Wt.	C	P	F
1 tsp. prepared mustard	5g	–	–	–
2 tbsp. cider vinegar	30g	–	–	–
1 tsp. salt	5g	–	–	–
dash pepper	–	–	–	–
1/4 tsp. oregano leaves, crushed	–	–	–	–
2 scallions, minced	35g	5	1	–
3 tbsp. pimiento, chopped	45g	5	1	–
1/2 cup Cheddar cheese (2 ounces), cut in 1/2" (1.25 cm) strips	60g	–	14	10
2 cups cooked rice	420g	90	12	–

Preparation: In a medium salad bowl, mix the first 6 ingredients well; add rest of ingredients and toss lightly.

Calories: 602 or 151 calories/serving

Servings: 4

Exchange Value:
1/2 meat exchange +
1 bread exchange +
1 10% vegetable exchange

Around-The-World Salads

Bean Sprouts, Chinese Specialty

Ingredients:	Wt.	C	P	F
4 cups raw bean sprouts	400g	20	4	–
2 tbsp. cider vinegar	30g	–	–	–
dash garlic powder	–	–	–	–
dash ground black pepper	–	–	–	–
1/2 tsp. sugar	2.5g	2.5	–	–
1/2 tsp. ground ginger	2.5g	–	–	–
1 tsp. salt	5g	–	–	–
2 tbsp. soya sauce	30g	–	–	–
1 tbsp. catsup	15g	–	–	–

Preparation: Cook sprouts according to directions on package; refrigerate. Combine rest of ingredients in a small casserole and heat until boiling point. Remove from heat and let cool. Pour over cooled bean sprouts and toss lightly.

Calories: 98 or 16 calories/serving
Servings: 6
Exchange Value: 1 5% vegetable exchange

Big Islands Salad

Ingredients:	Wt.	C	P	F
2 cups canned pineapple pieces, run under water and well-drained	500g	40	4	–
2 cups cooked rice, cold	420g	90	12	–
1/2 cup celery, chopped	64g	–	–	–
1/4 cup raisins	30g	20	2	–
1/4 cup dairy sour cream	60g	–	–	10
3 tbsp. dietetic mayonnaise	45g	–	–	5
1 tsp. salt	5g	–	–	–
1/4 tsp. ground ginger	–	–	–	–

Preparation: Combine pineapple pieces, rice, celery and raisins; toss lightly. Mix together well the rest of ingredients; pour them over rice mixture and toss again. Cover and refrigerate. Serve on lettuce bed.

Calories: 807 or 135 calories/serving
Servings: 6
Exchange Value: 1 bread exchange +
1 fruit exchange +
1/2 fat exchange

Canadian Mold

Ingredients:	Wt.	C	P	F
1 envelope unflavored gelatin	8g	–	–	–
1/4 cup cold water	50g	–	–	–
1 can (10 1/2 ounces) tomato soup, undiluted	300g	45	6	7.5
1/2 cup dairy sour cream	120g	–	–	20
1/2 cup celery, chopped	64g	–	–	–
3 tbsp. pimiento, chopped	45g	5	1	–
1 cup mild Canadian cheese (4 ounces) cubed	120g	–	28	20
2 hard-cooked eggs, chopped	100g	–	14	10

Preparation: Soften gelatin in cold water. Heat soup until boiling point; add gelatin and stir until dissolved. Let cool; add sour cream and celery. Refrigerate until partially set; then, fold in rest of ingredients. Pour into a 1 1/2 quart (1 5/8 litre) mold. Refrigerate until firm.

Calories: 914 or 152 calories/serving
Servings: 6
Exchange Value:

1 meat exchange +
1/2 bread exchange +
1 fat exchange

Chilean Salad

Ingredients:	Wt.	C	P	F
2 medium tomatoes, cut in pieces	180g	10	2	—
1 large green pepper, cut in 1/2" (1.25 cm) pieces	90g	7.5	1.5	—
1/4 cup celery, chopped	32g	—	—	—
1 scallion, minced	20g	—	—	—
2 bacon slices, crisply cooked, drained and crumbled	20g	—	—	10
2 hard-cooked eggs, sliced	100g	—	14	10
1/4 cup vinegar	60g	—	—	—
1/4 tsp. salt	—	—	—	—
1/4 tsp. chili powder	—	—	—	—

Preparation: Combine the first 6 ingredients. Heat vinegar, salt and chili powder to boiling point. Pour over vegetable mixture and toss.

Calories: 320 or 80 calories/serving

Servings: 4

Exchange Value: 1/2 meat exchange +
1 5% vegetable exchange +
1/2 fat exchange

Chinese Cucumber Salad

Ingredients:	Wt.	C	P	F
2 medium cucumbers	200g	20	4	–
1/4 cup creamy peanut butter	60g	–	14	30
1/4 cup cold water	50g	–	–	–
1/2 cup cooked chicken, cut in 1" (2.5 cm) strips	60g	–	14	10
1/2 tsp. salt	2.5g	–	–	–

Preparation: Peel cucumbers, cut them lengthwise and seed them. Then cut them diagonally in 1/4" (.625 cm) slices. Make a smooth paste with water and peanut butter; add chicken and salt. Set aside. When ready to use, mix together well cucumber slices and paste.

Calories: 568 or 142 calories/serving

Servings: 4

Exchange Value:
1 meat exchange +
1 5% vegetable exchange +
1 fat exchange

Chinese Delights

Ingredients:	Wt.	C	P	F
²/₃ cup uncooked rice	100g	90	12	–
1¹/₂ cups water	300g	–	–	–
1 small onion, minced	35g	5	1	–
2 tbsp. soya sauce	30g	–	–	–
1 small clove garlic, minced	–	–	–	–
2 cups cooked ham, diced	240g	–	56	40
¹/₂ cup celery, chopped	64g	–	–	–
3 ounces or 6 tbsp. dietetic mayonnaise	90g	–	–	10
1 tbsp. vinegar	15g	–	–	–
dash red pepper (cayenne)	–	–	–	–
³/₄ cup Swiss cheese, grated (3 ounces)	90g	–	21	15

Preparation: In a large skillet, cook rice over low heat until lightly browned. Add water, onion, soya sauce and garlic; mix well. Cover and cook for 20 minutes or until rice is tender and liquid absorbed. Add ham and celery; heat through. Add mayonnaise, vinegar, red pepper and cheese.

Calories: 1325 or 221 calories/serving
Servings: 6
Exchange Value: 2 meat exchanges + 1 bread exchange

Danish Delights

Ingredients:	Wt.	C	P	F
1 package (3 ounces) lemon flavored gelatin	85g	90	12	—
¾ cup boiling water	150g	—	—	—
2 cups creamed cottage cheese	480g	—	56	40
½ cup dairy sour cream	120g	—	—	20
4 ounces (1 cup) blue cheese, crumbled	120g	—	28	20
2 tsp. salt	10g	—	—	—
½ tsp. Worcestershire sauce	2.5g	—	—	—
½ tsp. lemon juice	2g	—	—	—
1 small scallion, minced	20g	—	—	—

Preparation: Dissolve gelatin in boiling water. In a large bowl, mix rest of ingredients, except scallion; beat with an electric mixer until very smooth, or as smooth as possible. Add gelatin and scallion. Pour into a 4-cup mold or 8 individual molds. Refrigerate until set.

Calories: 1464 or 183 calories/serving
Servings: 8
Exchange Value:

1 meat exchange +
1 5% vegetable exchange +
½ whole milk exchange (4 ounces)
        or
1½ meat exchanges +
1 10% vegetable exchange +
½ fat exchange

German Lettuce

Ingredients:	Wt.	C	P	F
3 bacon slices, diced	30g	–	–	15
1 tbsp. bacon fat	15g	–	–	15
1 egg, beaten	50g	–	7	5
1/4 cup vinegar	60g	–	–	–
1 small onion, minced	35g	5	1	–
non-caloric liquid sweetener to equal 2 tbsp. sugar	–	–	–	–
2 tbsp. water	25g	–	–	–
1/2 tsp. salt	2.5g	–	–	–
6 cups lettuce leaves, torn	420g	30	6	–

Preparation: In a medium skillet, fry bacon until crisp; drain all fat but 1 tbsp. Crumble bacon and set aside. Combine egg, vinegar, onion, non-caloric sweetener, water and salt; add to bacon and bacon fat. Heat until boiling point, stirring constantly. Heap lettuce in the bottom of a salad bowl and pour the hot dressing over it. Toss carefully.

Calories: 511 or 85 calories/serving
Servings: 6
Exchange Value: 1/2 bread exchange + 1 fat exchange

Hawaiian Salad

Ingredients:	Wt.	C	P	F
1 1/3 cups cooked, fresh, green peas	220g	40	4	—
1/2 tsp. salt	2.5g	—	—	—
1 tsp. curry powder	5g	—	—	—
1 1/2 cups unsweetened pineapple juice	320g	40	4	—
1 1/3 cups precooked rice	138g	120	16	—
dash pepper	—	—	—	—
1 1/4 cups cooked chicken, diced	150g	—	35	25
1/2 cup canned pineapple pieces, run under water and well-drained	125g	10	1	—
1/2 cup celery, chopped	64g	—	—	—
3/4 cup dietetic mayonnaise	180g	—	—	20

Preparation: Combine salt, curry powder and pineapple juice in a medium casserole; bring to boil. Add rice and stir well. Cover, remove from heat and let stand for 5 minutes. Add peas and pepper; mix lightly with a fork. Refrigerate. Just before serving, add rest of ingredients. Toss lightly.

Calories: 1485 or 248 calories/serving

Servings: 6

Exchange Value:
1 meat exchange +
2 bread exchanges +
1 5% vegetable exchange +
1/2 fat exchange

Honolulu Chicken

Ingredients:	Wt.	C	P	F
1 1/2 cups cooked chicken, cubed	180g	–	42	30
1 cup canned pineapple pieces, run under water and well-drained	250g	20	2	–
1/2 cup celery, finely chopped	64g	–	–	–
10 walnuts, finely chopped	14g	–	–	10
1/2 cup dairy sour cream	120g	–	–	20
3 tbsp. dietetic mayonnaise	45g	–	–	5

Preparation: Combine chicken, pineapple pieces, celery and nuts. Mix sour cream well with mayonnaise and pour over salad. Toss and refrigerate.

Calories: 841 or 210 calories/serving
Servings: 4
Exchange Value:

1 meat exchange +
1 fat exchange +
1/2 whole milk exchange (4 ounces)

Indian Salad

Ingredients:	Wt.	C	P	F
1 1/2 cups cooked ham, cut in 1" (2.5 cm) strips	180g	–	42	30
2 6" (15 cm) bananas, halved and cut in 1/2" (1.25 cm) slices	180g	40	4	–
40 peanuts	32g	–	–	20
3 tbsp. dietetic mayonnaise	45g	–	–	5
2 tbsp. lemon juice	25g	2.5	–	–
2 tbsp. milk	30g	1.5	1	1.25

Preparation: Combine ham, banana slices and peanuts. Toss lightly with the mixture of the other 3 ingredients.

Calories: 870 or 218 calories/serving

Servings: 4

Exchange Value: 1 1/2 meat exchanges +
1 fruit exchange +
1 1/2 fat exchanges

Italian Green Beans

Ingredients:	Wt.	C	P	F
1 package (10 ounces) frozen Italian green beans	188g	12.5	2.5	–
2 tbsp. butter or margarine	30g	–	–	30
3 bread slices, cubed	90g	45	6	–
1 cup whole kernel corn (cooked)	225g	45	6	–
3 ounces or 6 tbsp. dietetic mayonnaise	90g	–	–	10
2 tbsp. pimiento, chopped	30g	–	–	–
1/4 tsp. salt	–	–	–	–

Preparation: Cook beans according to directions; drain well and let cool. In a large skillet, melt fat; add bread cubes and brown until crisp, stirring occasionally. Mix beans, corn, mayonnaise, pimiento and salt. Refrigerate. Before serving, garnish salad with croutons and toss gently.

Calories: 828 or 104 calories/serving
Servings: 8
Exchange Value: 1/2 bread exchange +
1 5% vegetable exchange +
1 fat exchange

Italian Tomato Salad

Ingredients:	Wt.	C	P	F
6 medium tomatoes, ripe but firm	540g	30	6	–
1/8 tsp. garlic powder	–	–	–	–
1/2 tsp. salt	2.5g	–	–	–
1/2 tsp. sugar	2.5g	2.5	–	–
1/2 tsp. pepper	2.5g	–	–	–
1/2 tsp. oregano leaves, crushed	2.5g	–	–	–
1/2 tsp. basil leaves, crushed	2.5g	–	–	–
1 tsp. cider vinegar	5g	–	–	–
1 tbsp. salad oil	15g	–	–	15

Preparation: Wash tomatoes; do not peel. Cut them into 1" (2.5 cm) cubes and toss lightly with rest of ingredients. Refrigerate at least 30 minutes before serving.

Calories: 289 or 48 calories/serving
Servings: 6
Exchange Value: 1 5% vegetable exchange + 1/2 fat exchange

Neapolitan Salad

Ingredients:	Wt.	C	P	F
2 cups canned, cut, green beans, drained	300g	20	4	—
2 medium tomatoes, peeled, chopped and drained	180g	10	2	—
1 small onion, minced	35g	5	1	—
1/2 cup dairy sour cream	120g	—	—	20
2 tsp. salad oil	10g	—	—	10
1/2 tsp. vinegar	2.5g	—	—	—
dash garlic powder	—	—	—	—
dash salt and pepper	—	—	—	—
lettuce leaves	—	—	—	—

Preparation: Combine beans, tomatoes and onion. Mix together sour cream with rest of ingredients, except lettuce. Add to bean mixture and toss lightly. Refrigerate at least 2 hours before serving on lettuce leaves.

Calories: 438 or 73 calories/serving
Servings: 6
Exchange Value: 1 5% vegetable exchange +
1 fat exchange

Panama Chicken

Ingredients:	Wt.	C	P	F
2 medium cantaloups	1800g	40	4	–
2 cups cooked chicken, diced	240g	–	56	40
1/2 cup celery, chopped	64g	–	–	–
14 medium fresh green grapes, without seeds, halved	70g	10	1	–
5 small stuffed green olives, thinly sliced	45g	–	–	5
1/2 envelope dietetic topping for desserts "Dream Whip," prepared (1 cup)	–	19.2	3.2	–
3 tbsp. dietetic mayonnaise	45g	–	–	5

Preparation: Halve melons and remove seeds. Combine chicken, celery, grapes and olives; add 1/2 tsp. salt. Mix topping well with mayonnaise and pour this dressing over chicken salad. Toss gently but thoroughly. Spoon salad into melon cups. Refrigerate.

Calories: 984 or 246 calories/serving

Servings: 4

Exchange Value:
2 meat exchanges +
1/2 bread exchange +
1 fruit exchange +
1/2 fat exchange

Quebec Jelly

Ingredients:	Wt.	C	P	F
1 envelope unflavored gelatin	8g	–	–	–
3/4 cup cold water	150g	–	–	–
1 tsp. instant chicken broth powder or liquid base	5g	–	–	–
1 tsp. curry powder	5g	–	–	–
1 tbsp. lemon juice	12g	–	–	–
1/4 tsp. Worcestershire sauce	–	–	–	–
1 tsp. onion, grated	5g	–	–	–
1/2 tsp. salt	2.5g	–	–	–
1/4 cup dairy sour cream	60g	–	–	10
4 hard-cooked eggs, finely chopped	200g	–	28	20
1/2 cup cooked ham, ground	60g	–	14	10
1/2 cup celery, chopped	64g	–	–	–

Preparation: In a small casserole, soften gelatin in cold water; add instant chicken broth. Heat over low heat, stirring constantly, until gelatin and instant powder are dissolved. Add curry powder and mix well. Remove from heat; stir in lemon juice, Worcestershire sauce, onion and salt. Refrigerate until partially set. Then, slowly add to sour cream; fold in eggs, ham and celery. Pour into a 3-cup mold and refrigerate until firm.

Calories: 528 or 132 calories/serving
Servings: 4
Exchange Value: 1 1/2 meat exchanges + 1/2 fat exchange

Slav Salad

Ingredients:	Wt.	C	P	F
1/4 cup vinegar	60g	–	–	–
1 small clove garlic, crushed	–	–	–	–
1/2 tsp. salt	2.5g	–	–	–
1/4 tsp. pepper	–	–	–	–
7 cups raw cabbage, shredded	700g	70	14	–
3 medium cucumbers, unpeeled, sliced	300g	30	6	–
1 cup canned green peas, drained	180g	40	4	–
1 1/2 cups cooked beets, sliced	225g	30	3	–
1 cup cooked ham, cut in fine strips	120g	–	28	20
1 cup dairy sour cream	240g	–	–	40

Preparation: Mix together the first 4 ingredients. Pour over vegetables and ham; mix and let marinate for 1 hour. Just before serving, add sour cream and toss.

Calories: 1440 or 180 calories/serving

Servings: 8

Exchange Value:

1/2 meat exchange +
1 1/2 bread exchanges +
1 fat exchange
       or
1 bread exchange +
1/2 fat exchange +
1/2 whole milk exchange (4 ounces)

Fruit Salads

Apple Salad

Ingredients:	Wt.	C	P	F
4 medium apples, unpeeled and diced	600g	80	8	—
4 ounces (1 cup) Swiss cheese or Cheddar cheese, cubed	120g	—	28	20
1/2 cup celery, chopped	64g	—	—	—
1/2 cup dairy sour cream	120g	—	—	20
dash salt	—	—	—	—

Preparation: Combine all ingredients and refrigerate a few hours before serving.

Calories: 824 or 137 calories/serving
Servings: 6
Exchange Value: 1/2 meat exchange +
1 bread exchange +
1/2 fat exchange

Fruited Melon

Ingredients:	Wt.	C	P	F
1 cup watermelon cubes	150g	10	1	—
1 medium fresh peach, diced	95g	10	1	—
½ cup canned pineapple pieces, run under water and well-drained	125g	10	1	—
2 tbsp. white sugar	30g	30	4	—
3 ounces unsweetened pineapple juice	80g	10	1	—
3 tbsp. dietetic mayonnaise	45g	—	—	5
1 envelope dietetic topping for desserts "Dream Whip," prepared (2 cups)	—	38.4	6.4	—

Preparation: Mix fruits lightly and refrigerate. Mix sugar, pineapple juice and mayonnaise together well. Fold in fruits, then topping. Pour into a 4-cup mold and refrigerate until set.

Calories: 536 or 89 calories/serving
Servings: 6
Exchange
Value:

2 fruit exchanges
or
1 bread exchange +
1 5% vegetable exchange
or
1 10% vegetable exchange +
1 fruit exchange

Garnished Fruit Salad

Ingredients:	Wt.	C	P	F
1½ cups canned pineapple pieces, run under water and well-drained	225g	30	3	–
1 cup small cantaloup balls	200g	10	1	–
1 cup small watermelon balls	150g	10	1	–
1 medium fresh peach, cut in strips*	95g	10	1	–
1½ tbsp. white sugar	22g	22.5	3	–
½ cup heavy cream (35%), whipped	120g	–	–	40

Preparation: Combine all fruits in a large bowl. Sprinkle with sugar, then fold in whipped cream. Refrigerate a few hours before serving on lettuce.

Calories: 726 or 121 calories/serving

Servings: 6

Exchange Value:

1 bread exchange +
1 fat exchange

*Dip in lemon juice diluted with water to prevent discoloration.

Irresistible Fruit Salad

Ingredients:	Wt.	C	P	F
24 fresh green grapes, without seeds	140g	20	2	—
1 cup canned pineapple pieces, run under water and well-drained	250g	20	2	—
1 cup orange quarters, diced	200g	20	2	—
1 cup cantaloup balls	200g	10	1	—
20 big red cherries	150g	20	1	—
2 medium plums, sliced	80g	10	1	—

Salad dressing:

	Wt.	C	P	F
2 eggs, beaten	100g	—	14	10
2 tbsp. unsweetened orange juice	25g	2.5	—	—
2 tbsp. vinegar	30g	—	—	—
non-caloric liquid sweetener to equal 1/4 cup sugar	—	—	—	—
dash salt	—	—	—	—
1 cup dairy sour cream	240g	—	—	40

Preparation: Combine all fruits, then pour salad dressing over. Refrigerate at least 24 hours before serving.
Salad dressing: In a small casserole, combine eggs, orange juice, vinegar, sweetener and salt. Cook over low heat, stirring constantly, until sauce thickens. Remove from heat. Let cool, then add sour cream. Refrigerate.

Calories: 956 or 120 calories/serving
Servings: 8
Exchange Value:
1/2 bread exchange +
1/2 whole milk exchange (4 ounces)
          or
1 bread exchange +
1 fat exchange

Fruit-Dessert Molded Salads

Cheese and Grapefruit Jelly

Ingredients:	Wt.	C	P	F
2 envelopes unflavored gelatin	16g	–	–	–
1/2 cup cold water	100g	–	–	–
1 cup boiling water	200g	–	–	–
non-caloric liquid sweetener to equal 1/3 cup sugar	–	–	–	–
3/4 tsp. salt	3.75g	–	–	–
2 cups grapefruit quarters	400g	40	4	–
1/4 cup unsweetened orange juice	50g	5	.5	–
1 package (6 ounces) cream cheese, softened	180g	–	–	60
2 tbsp. water	25g	–	–	–
1 tbsp. sugar	15g	15	2	–
dash salt	–	–	–	–

Preparation: Soften gelatin in cold water; add boiling water and stir until dissolved. Add sweetener, 3/4 tsp. salt, grapefruit quarters and orange juice. Pour half of this mixture into a 6-cup mold and refrigerate until firm. Beat cream cheese with water, sugar and dash salt; spread this cream on firm gelatin. Carefully, pour rest of gelatin over cheese and refrigerate until set.

Calories: 806 or 134 calories/serving
Servings: 6
Exchange Value: 1 fruit exchange +
2 fat exchanges

Cheesy Pineapple Salad

Ingredients:	Wt.	C	P	F
1 cup canned, crushed pineapple, run under water and well-drained	250g	20	2	–
1/4 cup cold water	50g	–	–	–
1/2 cup boiling water	100g	–	–	–
1 tbsp. lemon juice	12g	–	–	–
non-caloric liquid sweetener to equal 1/2 cup sugar	–	–	–	–
1 envelope unflavored gelatin	8g	–	–	–
3/4 cup Cheddar cheese, grated (3 ounces)	90g	–	21	15
1 envelope dietetic topping for desserts "Dream Whip," prepared (2 cups)	–	38.4	6.4	–

Preparation: Mix pineapple, lemon juice and sweetener. Soften gelatin in cold water; add boiling water and stir until dissolved. Pour over pineapple and refrigerate until almost firm. Fold in cheese and topping. Refrigerate until set.

Calories: 486 or 81 calories/serving
Servings: 6
Exchange Value: 1/2 meat exchange +
1 fruit exchange

Cocktail in Aspic

Ingredients:	Wt.	C	P	F
1 envelope unflavored gelatin	8g	–	–	–
2 cups unsweetened white grape juice	440g	80	8	–
28 fresh green grapes, halved	140g	20	2	–
1 cup canned crushed pineapple, run under water and well-drained	125g	10	1	–
3/8 cup dairy sour cream	90g	–	–	15

Preparation: In a medium casserole, soften gelatin in 1 cup grape juice. Heat over low heat, stirring constantly, until dissolved. Add rest of grape juice and refrigerate until partially set. Fold in rest of ingredients and pour into a 4-cup mold. Refrigerate until firm.

Calories: 619 or 103 calories/serving

Servings: 6

Exchange Value:

1/2 bread exchange +
1 fruit exchange +
1/2 fat exchange

Fruit and Cheese Canapés

Ingredients:	Wt.	C	P	F
2 cups unsweetened applesauce	400g	40	4	–
1 package (3 ounces) pineapple flavored gelatin	85g	90	12	–
1 tbsp. fresh lemon juice	12g	–	–	–
1 envelope unflavored gelatin	8g	–	–	–
1¹/₂ cups creamed cottage cheese, well-drained	360g	–	42	30
2 ounces cream cheese, softened	60g	–	–	20
¹/₂ cup celery, diced	64g	–	–	–

Preparation: Heat applesauce with ²/₃ cup water until boiling point. Add flavored gelatin and lemon juice; stir until dissolved. Let cool. Set aside half of this mixture and pour the other half into a 8¹/₂"×4¹/₂"×2¹/₂" (21.25 cm×11.25 cm×6.25 cm) dish. Refrigerate until almost firm. In a medium casserole, soften unflavored gelatin in ¹/₂ cup water; stir over low heat until dissolved. With cottage cheese and cream cheese, make a paste as smooth as possible; slowly stir in unflavored gelatin and celery and mix well. Pour over almost firm gelatin, then refrigerate until the mixture is almost firm again. Then, pour remaining applesauce mixture over the cheese layer. Refrigerate until set. Cut in squares.

Calories: 1202 or 150 calories/serving

Servings: 8

Exchange Value:
1 meat exchange +
1 bread exchange
    or
¹/₂ bread exchange +
¹/₂ fruit exchange +
¹/₂ whole milk exchange (4 ounces)

Grass-Land Salad

Ingredients:	Wt.	C	P	F
1 package (3 ounces) lime flavored gelatin	85g	90	12	—
1 cup boiling water	200g	—	—	—
1 envelope unflavored gelatin	8g	—	—	—
1/4 cup cold water	50g	—	—	—
1 cup dietetic ginger ale	208g	—	—	—
1 1/2 cups creamed cottage cheese, well-drained	360g	—	42	30

Preparation: Dissolve flavored gelatin in boiling water. Soften unflavored gelatin in cold water; add to flavored gelatin and stir until well dissolved. Slowly stir in ginger ale. Refrigerate until partially set; then fold in cottage cheese. Pour into a 3 1/2-cup mold. Refrigerate until firm.

Calories: 846 or 141 calories/serving

Servings: 6

Exchange Value: 1 meat exchange +
1 bread exchange

Jellied Cocktail

Ingredients:	Wt.	C	P	F
2 cups canned fruit salad, run under water and well-drained	435g	30	3	–
1 package (3 ounces) lime flavored gelatin	85g	90	12	–
3/4 cup dietetic ginger ale	156g	–	–	–
3/4 cup boiling water	150g	–	–	–

Preparation: Dissolve gelatin in boiling water; add ginger ale. Refrigerate until partially set; then fold in well-drained fruits. Pour into a 3½-cup mold. Refrigerate until firm.

Calories: 540 or 108 calories/serving
Servings: 5
Exchange Value: 1 bread exchange +
1 fruit exchange

Jellied Waldorf Salad

Ingredients:	Wt.	C	P	F
1 envelope unflavored gelatin	8g	–	–	–
1 package (3 ounces) lemon flavored gelatin	85g	90	12	–
1 cup boiling water	200g	–	–	–
2 cups buttermilk	480g	24	16	–
1 medium red apple, finely chopped	150g	20	2	–
1 cup celery, chopped	128g	2.5	.5	–
20 walnuts, chopped	28g	–	–	20
3 ounces or 6 tbsp. dietetic mayonnaise	90g	–	–	10
3/4 cup dairy sour cream	180g	–	–	30

Preparation: In a large mixing bowl, combine gelatins. Add boiling water and stir until both are well dissolved. Add buttermilk and refrigerate until slightly thickened. Meanwhile, mix rest of ingredients well; fold in thickened gelatin and mix well. Pour into a 6-cup, crown-form mold. Refrigerate until set.

Calories: 1208 or 151 calories/serving

Servings: 8

Exchange Value:

1/2 meat exchange +
1 bread exchange +
1 fat exchange
            or
1/2 bread exchange +
1 10% vegetable exchange +
1 1/2 fat exchanges

Little Fruited Cheese Molds

Ingredients:	Wt.	C	P	F
1 package (3 ounces) pineapple flavored gelatin	85g	90	12	—
1 cup unsweetened orange juice	200g	20	2	—
1/2 envelope dietetic topping for desserts "Dream Whip," prepared (1 cup)	—	19.2	3.2	—
1 package (3 ounces) cream cheese, softened	90g	—	—	30
1/8 tsp. ground allspice	—	—	—	—
1/8 tsp. ground nutmeg	—	—	—	—
1 cup dietetic ginger ale	208g	—	—	—

Preparation: Heat orange juice with spices until boiling point; add gelatin and stir until dissolved. Add ginger ale. Refrigerate until partially set. Mix small amount of topping with cream cheese and make a paste as smooth as possible. Add rest of topping and fold into partially-set gelatin. Pour into 6 individual molds. Refrigerate until firm.

Calories: 856 or 143 calories/serving
Servings: 6
Exchange Value: 1 1/2 bread exchanges +
1 fat exchange

Orange Salad-Dessert

Ingredients:	Wt.	C	P	F
6 canned, big, peach halves, run under water and well-drained, sliced	465g	30	3	—
3/4 cup cold water	150g	—	—	—
2 packages (3 ounces each) orange flavored gelatin	170g	180	24	—
2 cups boiling water	400g	—	—	—
10 walnuts, chopped	14g	—	—	10
2 cups vanilla ice cream	228g	45	6	30
1 6" (15 cm) banana, peeled and sliced	90g	20	2	—

Preparation: Dissolve gelatin in boiling water. To half of this mixture, add 3/4 cup cold water and refrigerate until partially set; then fold in peach slices and nuts. Pour into a 6 1/2-cup mold; refrigerate until almost firm. Meanwhile, melt ice cream in the other gelatin-half mixture; refrigerate until partially set, then fold in sliced banana. Pour carefully over the gelatin-peach layer. Refrigerate until firm.

Calories: 1600 or 133 calories/serving
Servings: 12
Exchange Value:

1 1/2 bread exchanges +
1/2 fat exchange
            or
2 fruit exchanges +
1/4 whole milk exchange (2 ounces)

Orchard Salad

Ingredients:	Wt.	C	P	F
1 package (3 ounces) lemon flavored gelatin	85g	90	12	–
³/₄ cup unsweetened apple juice, heated to boiling point	170g	20	2	–
³/₄ cup cold unsweetened apple juice	170g	20	2	–
1 medium apple, unpeeled and chopped	150g	20	2	–
10 walnuts, chopped	14g	–	–	10
1 envelope dietetic topping for desserts "Dream Whip," prepared (2 cups)	–	38.4	6.4	–

Preparation: Dissolve gelatin in almost boiling apple juice; add cold apple juice and refrigerate until partially set. To half of this mixture, add apple and nuts; pour into a 5½-cup mold. Refrigerate until almost firm. Fold topping into the other half of the gelatin mixture. Pour over first layer in the mold. Refrigerate until set.

Calories: 941 or 157 calories/serving
Servings: 6
Exchange Value:

1 bread exchange +
1 fruit exchange +
½ skimmed milk exchange (4 ounces)
        or
1½ bread exchanges
1 fruit exchange

Refrigerated Rhubarb Salad

Ingredients:	Wt.	C	P	F
1 cup fresh rhubarb, diced	120g	5	.5	–
2 tbsp. water	25g	–	–	–
non-caloric liquid sweetener to equal ¼ cup sugar	–	–	–	–
1 cup canned crushed pineapple, run under water and well-drained	250g	20	2	–
1 package (8 ounces) cream cheese, softened	240g	–	–	80
non-caloric liquid sweetener to equal ¼ cup sugar	–	–	–	–
1 tbsp. lemon juice	12g	–	–	–
7 drops red food color	–	–	–	–
3 ounces unsweetened pineapple juice	80g	10	1	–
1 envelope dietetic topping for desserts "Dream Whip," prepared (2 cups)	–	38.4	6.4	–

Preparation: In a small casserole, combine rhubarb, water and sweetener (to equal ¼ cup sugar). Cover and cook over medium heat, stirring occasionally, for 3 minutes or until rhubarb is tender; let cool. Then, mix pineapple with rhubarb. Beat cream cheese, sweetener (to equal ¼ cup sugar), lemon juice, food color and pineapple juice; fold in fruits and topping. Pour into 8 individual molds. Refrigerate until firm.

Calories: 1054 or 132 calories/serving
Servings: 8
Exchange Value: 1 fruit exchange +
2 fat exchanges

Spiced Molded Duet

Ingredients:	Wt.	C	P	F
8 canned peach halves, run under water and well-drained	620g	40	4	–
1 1/2 cups unsweetened orange juice	300g	30	3	–
1/2 tsp. whole cloves	–	–	–	–
1 2" (5 cm) cinnamon stick	–	–	–	–
1/4 cup vinegar	60g	–	–	–
1 package (3 ounces) lemon flavored gelatin	85g	90	12	–
1 cup fresh cranberries	113g	13	.5	.6
non-caloric liquid sweetener to equal 1/3 cup sugar	–	–	–	–
1 3/4 cups hot water	350g	–	–	–
1 package (3 ounces) cherry flavored gelatin	85g	90	12	–

Preparation: To orange juice add spices and vinegar; heat and let simmer for 10 minutes. Add peaches and heat over low heat for 5 minutes. Remove peaches from juice and put in a crown-form mold of 2 quarts (2 1/4 litres). The round side of the peaches must touch the bottom of the mold, not the halved section. Remove cloves and cinnamon stick from juice; measure juice and, if necessary, add enough water to make 1 3/4 cups liquid. Add this liquid to lemon gelatin and stir until perfectly dissolved. Pour over peaches and refrigerate until almost firm. Meanwhile, finely chop cranberries; add sweetener and set aside. Add hot water to cherry gelatin and stir until well dissolved. Let cool, then add to cranberry mixture. Pour over almost-firm peach layer and refrigerate until firm.

Exchange Value:
1 bread exchange +
1 fruit exchange

Calories: 1183 or 118 calories/serving
Servings: 10

Supreme Grapes Salad

Ingredients:	Wt.	C	P	F
1 envelope unflavored gelatin	8g	—	—	—
1/4 cup cold water	50g	—	—	—
1 cup boiling water	200g	—	—	—
non-caloric liquid sweetener to equal 1/3 cup sugar	—	—	—	—
dash salt	—	—	—	—
1 can (6 ounces) frozen concentrated grape juice, unsweetened, thawed	180g	120	12	—
2 tbsp. fresh lemon juice	25g	2.5	—	—
28 fresh green grapes, halved	140g	20	2	—
2 6" (15 cm) bananas, peeled and diced	180g	40	4	—

Preparation: Soften gelatin in cold water; add boiling water, non-caloric sweetener and salt. Stir until gelatin is dissolved. Add grape juice and lemon juice. Refrigerate until partially set. Fold in fruits. Pour into 6 individual molds. Refrigerate until firm.

Calories: 802 or 134 calories/serving
Servings: 6
Exchange Value: 2 bread exchanges

Sweety Fruits

Ingredients:	Wt.	C	P	F
1 package (3 ounces) lime flavored gelatin	85g	90	12	–
3/4 cup dietetic lemon beverage	156g	–	–	–
1 cup canned crushed pineapple, run under water and well-drained	250g	20	2	–
1/2 envelope dietetic topping for desserts "Dream Whip," (1 cup)	–	19.2	3.2	–
1/4 cup Cheddar cheese, grated (1 ounce)	30g	–	7	5

Preparation: Dissolve gelatin in 3/4 cup boiling water; slowly, stir in lemon beverage. Refrigerate until partially set; then fold in pineapple, topping and cheese. Pour into 6 individual molds. Refrigerate until firm.

Calories: 659 or 110 calories/serving
Servings: 6
Exchange Value: 1 bread exchange +
1/2 skimmed milk exchange (4 ounces)

Sauces and Salad Dressings

All-Purpose Sauce

Ingredients:	Wt.	C	P	F
1 tbsp. cornstarch	8g	7.5	1	–
1/2 tsp. dry mustard	2.5g	–	–	–
1 cup cold water	200g	–	–	–
1/4 cup vinegar	60g	–	–	–
1/4 cup catsup	60g	17	2	–
1/2 tsp. paprika	2.5g	–	–	–
1/2 tsp. horseradish	2.5g	–	–	–
1/2 tsp. Worcestershire sauce	2.5g	–	–	–
dash salt	–	–	–	–
1 tsp. sugar	5g	5	.6	–
1 garlic clove, halved	–	–	–	–

Preparation: Combine cornstarch and mustard in a small saucepan. Gradually, stir in cold water. Cook over medium heat, stirring constantly, until sauce thickens. Let cool. Add remaining ingredients except garlic. Beat until smooth. Add garlic, cover and refrigerate. Shake well before using. Wonderful with green salads.

Yielding: 1 1/2 cups
Calories: 132
Exchange Value: 2 tbsp. = free food if taken in this proportion
= 11 calories

Banana Sauce

Ingredients:	Wt.	C	P	F
1 3-ounce package cream cheese, softened	90g	–	–	30
2 tbsp. milk	30g	1.5	1	1.25
1 6" (15 cm) banana, ripe	90g	20	2	–
1 tbsp. granulated sugar	15g	15	2	–
1 tbsp. fresh lemon juice	12g	–	–	–
dash salt	–	–	–	–

Preparation: Make a cream as smooth as possible with cream cheese and milk. Mash banana and add sugar, lemon juice and salt. Thoroughly mix cream cheese mixture with banana mixture. Serve with fruit salads.

Yielding: 1 cup

Calories: 447

Exchange Value:

3 tbsp. = ½ bread exchange +
1 fat exchange
= 84 calories

Coleslaw Dressing

Ingredients:	Wt.	C	P	F
1/4 cup dairy sour cream	60g	–	–	10
1/4 cup vinegar	60g	–	–	–
4 tsp. sugar	20g	20	2.6	–
1/2 tsp. salt	2.5g	–	–	–
dash pepper	–	–	–	–

Preparation: Beat all ingredients well and refrigerate.

Yielding: 1/2 cup
Calories: 180
Exchange Value:

2 tbsp. = 1 5% vegetable exchange +
1/2 fat exchange
= 45 calories
1 tbsp. = 1/2 5% vegetable exchange +
1/4 fat exchange
= 23 calories

Coleslaw Sauce

Ingredients:	Wt.	C	P	F
³/₄ cup evaporated milk	180g	18	12	15
¹/₄ cup vinegar	60g	–	–	–
non-caloric liquid sweetener to equal ¹/₄ cup sugar	–	–	–	–
1 egg	50g	–	7	5
1 tsp. celery salt	5g	–	–	–
1 tsp. salt	5g	–	–	–
dash pepper	–	–	–	–

Preparation: Beat ingredients until very smooth. Pour into a saucepan and cook, stirring constantly, until sauce thickens. Refrigerate.

Yielding: 1 cup
Calories: 328
**Exchange
Value:** 2 tbsp. = ¹/₄ whole milk exchange (2 ounces)
  = 41 calories

Coleslaw Sauce, Old Style

Ingredients:	Wt.	C	P	F
1/2 cup buttermilk	120g	6	4	—
1/4 cup vinegar	60g	—	—	—
1 1/2 tsp. cornstarch	4g	3.75	.5	—
1 egg yolk	17g	—	3	5
1/2 tsp. onion salt	2.5g	—	—	—
1/4 tsp. dry mustard	—	—	—	—
1 tbsp. sugar	15g	15	2	—
1 tsp. caraway seeds	5g	—	—	—
dash pepper	—	—	—	—

Preparation: In a small saucepan, bring buttermilk to boiling point, stirring constantly. Remove from heat and slowly add cornstarch, well diluted in vinegar. Cook, stirring constantly, until mixture begins to boil. Remove from heat and beat egg yolk into mixture; add remaining ingredients and refrigerate.

Yielding: 3/4 cup
Calories: 182
Exchange Value:

2 tbsp. = 1 5% vegetable exchange
= 30 calories

Cooked Sauce

Ingredients:	Wt.	C	P	F
2 tbsp. flour	14g	12	1.6	–
2 tbsp. sugar	30g	30	4	–
1 tsp. salt	5g	–	–	–
1 tsp. mustard (dry)	5g	–	–	–
2 egg yolks, lightly beaten	34g	–	6	10
3/4 cup milk	180g	9	6	7.5
1/4 cup vinegar	60g	–	–	–
1 tsp. butter or margarine	5g	–	–	5

Preparation: Combine flour, sugar and mustard in a double boiler. Add egg yolks and milk; cook over very hot water (not boiling), stirring constantly, until thickened. Add vinegar and fat. Let cool.

Yielding: 1 cup
Calories: 477
Exchange Value: 2 tbsp. = 1/2 bread exchange +
1/2 fat exchange
= 60 calories

Cottage Cheese Sauce

Ingredients:	Wt.	C	P	F
2 tbsp. lemon juice	25g	2.5	–	–
1/2 cup creamed cottage cheese	120g	–	14	10
3 ounces evaporated milk, undiluted	90g	9	6	7.5
1/2 tsp. salt	2.5g	–	–	–
non-caloric liquid sweetener to equal 2 tsp. sugar	–	–	–	–
dash paprika	–	–	–	–

Preparation: Beat together all ingredients until smooth.

Yielding: 1 cup
Calories: 284
Exchange
Value: 2 tbsp. = 1/2 meat exchange
                = 36 calories

Curry Sauce

Ingredients:	Wt.	C	P	F
3/4 cup plain yogurt	180g	12	8	5
2 tsp. prepared mustard	10g	–	–	–
1/2 tsp. salt	2.5g	–	–	–
1/2 tsp. curry powder	2.5g	–	–	–
minced parsley	–	–	–	–

Preparation: Mix the first 4 ingredients well. Sprinkle top with parsley and refrigerate. Delicious with green salads, especially with spinach or with broccoli.

Yielding: 3/4 cup
Calories: 125
Exchange Value: 2 tbsp. = 1/4 skim milk exchange (2 ounces)
= 21 calories

Emergency Sauce

Ingredients:	Wt.	C	P	F
3/4 cup water	150g	–	–	–
2 tsp. cornstarch	5g	5	.6	–
1/4 cup lemon juice	50g	5	.5	–
3/4 tsp. salt	3.75g	–	–	–
1 tsp. sugar	5g	5	.6	–
1/2 tsp. horseradish	2.5g	–	–	–
1 tsp. prepared mustard	5g	–	–	–
1/2 tsp. paprika	2.5g	–	–	–
1/2 tsp. Worcestershire sauce	2.5g	–	–	–
1/4 cup catsup	60g	17	2	–

Preparation: Dilute cornstarch in water; heat over low heat, stirring constantly, until mixture thickens. Let cool. Add remaining ingredients; beat with a mixer until very smooth. Refrigerate. Shake well before using.

Yielding: 1 1/4 cups
Calories: 141
Exchange Value: 2 tbsp. = free food if taken in this proportion
= 14 calories

English Sauce

Ingredients:	Wt.	C	P	F
2 tbsp. wine vinegar	30g	–	–	–
1 tsp. sugar	5g	5	.6	–
1 tsp. dry mustard	5g	–	–	–
1/2 tsp. salt	2.5g	–	–	–
dash pepper	–	–	–	–

Preparation: Mix all ingredients well.

Yielding: 3 tbsp.
Calories: 22
Exchange Value: 1 tbsp. = free food if taken in this proportion
= 7 calories

Exotic Sauce

Ingredients:	Wt.	C	P	F
3/4 cup unsweetened pineapple juice	160g	20	2	—
1/4 cup catsup	60g	17	2	—
2 tbsp. lemon juice	25g	2.5	—	—
1 small scallion, minced	20g	—	—	—
2 tsp. soya sauce	10g	—	—	—
dash pepper	—	—	—	—

Preparation: Mix all ingredients well and refrigerate. Serve with fruit or seafood salads.

Yielding: 1 cup
Calories: 174
Exchange Value:

2 tbsp. = 1 5% vegetable exchange
= 22 calories

French Sauce

Ingredients:	Wt.	C	P	F
1/2 cup water	100g	—	—	—
1/2 cup wine vinegar	120g	—	—	—
2 tsp. cornstarch	5g	5	.6	—
1 tbsp. lemon juice	12g	—	—	—
1/4 tsp. paprika	—	—	—	—
1/4 tsp. dry mustard	—	—	—	—
1 tsp. salt	5g	—	—	—
2 tbsp. catsup	30g	—	—	—
dash pepper	—	—	—	—

Preparation: Bring water and vinegar to boiling point. Remove from heat; add cornstarch, well diluted in lemon juice. Cook over low heat, stirring constantly, until sauce begins to boil. Remove from heat. Add remaining ingredients and beat until smooth. Let cool before refrigerating.

Yielding: 1 cup
Calories: 22
Exchange Value: 2 tbsp. = free food
= 3 calories

Fresh Sauce

Ingredients:	Wt.	C	P	F
3/4 cup dairy sour cream	180g	–	–	30
1/4 cup lemon juice	50g	5	.5	–
1/2 tsp. salt	2.5g	–	–	–
3 tbsp. pimiento, finely chopped	45g	5	1	–
1 tbsp. sugar	15g	15	2	–

Preparation: Mix all ingredients together well and refrigerate.

Yielding: 1 1/4 cups
Calories: 384
**Exchange
Value:**

2 tbsp. = 1/2 5% vegetable exchange +
1/2 fat exchange
= 38 calories

Fruit Salad Sauce

Ingredients:	Wt.	C	P	F
1 garlic clove, minced	–	–	–	–
1/4 cup vinegar	60g	–	–	–
1/2 cup unsweetened orange juice	100g	10	1	–
1 tsp. sugar	5g	5	.6	–
1/2 tsp. salt	2.5g	–	–	–

Preparation: Let garlic steep in vinegar for 1 hour, then strain. To vinegar, add remaining ingredients and shake well. Refrigerate. Shake again before using.

Yielding: 3/4 cup
Calories: 66
Exchange Value: 2 tbsp. = free food if taken in this proportion
= 11 calories

Garnishing Sauce

Ingredients:	Wt.	C	P	F
1/2 cup plain yogurt	120g	8	5.3	3.3
1/4 cup creamed cottage cheese	60g	–	7	5
1 tbsp. white granulated sugar	15g	15	2	–

Preparation: Mix all ingredients well. Serve on fruit salad. Especially delicious with pears.

Yielding: 3/4 cup
Calories: 224
Exchange Value: 2 tbsp. = 1/4 whole milk exchange (2 ounces)
= 37 calories

Grapefruit Sauce

Ingredients:	Wt.	C	P	F
1 cup unsweetened grapefruit juice	200g	20	2	–
1 tbsp. cornstarch	8g	7.5	1	–
1 tbsp. lemon juice	12g	–	–	–
1 tsp. honey	5g	5	.6	–
1/8 tsp. ground cloves	–	–	–	–
1/2 tsp. ground cinnamon	2.5g	–	–	–
1/4 tsp. ground ginger	–	–	–	–
1/2 tsp. salt	2.5g	–	–	–

Preparation: In a small saucepan, bring grapefruit juice to boiling point. Remove from heat and add cornstarch, well diluted in lemon juice. Cook over low heat, stirring constantly, until mixture begins to boil. Remove from heat and add remaining ingredients. Stir vigorously and refrigerate. Wonderful with fruit salads or on lettuce hearts.

Yielding: 1 1/4 cups
Calories: 144
Exchange Value: 2 tbsp. = free food if taken in this proportion
= 14 calories

Honey Fragrance Sauce

Ingredients:

Ingredients:	Wt.	C	P	F
1/2 cup dairy sour cream	120g	–	–	20
1 tbsp. honey	21g	15	2	–
1 tsp. fresh lemon juice	4g	–	–	–
dash salt	–	–	–	–

Preparation: Combine all ingredients; mix well and refrigerate. Serve with canned fruits or with fruit salads.

Yielding: 1/2 cup
Calories: 248
Exchange Value:

2 tbsp. = 1/2 fruit exchange +
1 fat exchange
= 62 calories

Lemon French Sauce

Ingredients:	Wt.	C	P	F
1 tsp. unflavored gelatin	2.6g	–	–	–
1 tbsp. cold water	12g	–	–	–
1/4 cup boiling water	50g	–	–	–
2 tbsp. sugar	30g	30	4	–
1/2 tsp. salt	2.5g	–	–	–
1 tsp. fresh lemon peel, grated	5g	–	–	–
1/2 cup fresh lemon juice	100g	10	1	–
1/4 tsp. garlic salt	–	–	–	–
dash pepper	–	–	–	–
1/8 tsp. dry mustard	–	–	–	–
1/4 tsp. Worcestershire sauce	–	–	–	–

Preparation: Soften gelatin in cold water; add boiling water and stir until dissolved. Add sugar and salt and stir again until completely dissolved. Combine this mixture with remaining ingredients in a jar with an air-tight lid; cover and shake well. Refrigerate. When ready to serve, soak jar in hot water for a few seconds so as to liquify gelatin. Serve with a green salad.

Yielding: 1 cup
Calories: 180
Exchange Value: 2 tbsp. = 1 5% vegetable exchange
= 23 calories

Lemon Sauce

Ingredients:	Wt.	C	P	F
3/4 cup water	150g	—	—	—
1 tbsp. cornstarch	8g	7.5	1	—
2 tbsp. lemon juice	25g	2.5	—	—
1/2 tsp. salt	2.5g	—	—	—
2 tsp. sugar	10g	10	1.3	—
2 tbsp. dairy sour cream	30g	—	—	5
dash pepper	—	—	—	—

Preparation: In a small saucepan, bring water to boiling point. Remove from heat and add cornstarch, well diluted in lemon juice. Cook over low heat, stirring constantly, until mixture begins to boil. Remove from heat and add remaining ingredients. Refrigerate. Excellent with potato salads, fruit salads or vegetable salads.

Yielding: 1 cup
Calories: 134
Exchange Value: 2 tbsp. = 1/2 5% vegetable exchange
= 17 calories

Fruited Sauce

Ingredients:	Wt.	C	P	F
1 small garlic clove, minced	–	–	–	–
1/4 cup vinegar	60g	–	–	–
1/2 cup unsweetened orange juice	100g	10	1	–
1/4 tsp. paprika	–	–	–	–
1 tsp. sugar	5g	5	.6	–
1/2 tsp. salt	2.5g	–	–	–

Preparation: Let garlic steep in vinegar for 1 hour, then strain. Add remaining ingredients and shake well. Refrigerate. Shake before using.

Yielding: 3/4 cup

Calories: 66

Exchange Value:

2 tbsp. = 1/2 5% vegetable exchange

or

free food if taken in this proportion

= 11 calories

Lightly Cheesy Sauce

Ingredients:	Wt.	C	P	F
1/2 cup cottage cheese, creamed	120g	–	14	10
2 tbsp. lemon juice	25g	2.5	1	–
1/4 cup evaporated milk, undiluted	60g	6	4	5
1/2 tsp. salt	2.5g	–	–	–
2 tsp. sugar	10g	10	1.2	–
2 tsp. onion, minced or grated	10g	–	–	–

Preparation: Mix all ingredients well.

Yielding: 7 ounces
Calories: 286
Exchange Value: 2 tbsp. = 1/4 whole milk exchange (2 ounces)
       = 41 calories

Mayonnaise

Ingredients:	Wt.	C	P	F
3 tbsp. sugar	45g	45	6	–
1 1/2 tsp. salt	7.5g	–	–	–
1 1/2 tsp. dry mustard	7.5g	–	–	–
2 eggs	100g	–	14	10
1 tbsp. cornstarch	8g	7.5	1	–
dash paprika	–	–	–	–
dash red pepper	–	–	–	–
1/2 cup milk	120g	6	4	5
1/2 cup vinegar	120g	–	–	–
1 tbsp. butter or margarine	15g	–	–	15

Preparation: Break eggs in a double boiler; sprinkle them with sugar, salt, mustard, cornstarch, paprika and red pepper. Beat strenuously with a rotary beater until very smooth. Stir in milk and cook over boiling water, stirring constantly, until sauce thickens. Slowly, add vinegar, continue cooking for 10 minutes, stirring once in a while. Remove from heat; add fat and mix well. Pour into a jar; do not cover before sauce is very cold.

Yielding: 1 1/4 cups
Calories: 604
Exchange Value:

2 tbsp. = 1/2 meat exchange +
     1 5% vegetable exchange
   = 60 calories

Mushroom Sauce

Ingredients:	Wt.	C	P	F
½ cup canned mushrooms, drained and chopped	60g	–	–	–
1 cup dairy sour cream	240g	–	–	40
3 tbsp. dietetic mayonnaise	45g	–	–	5
1 dill pickle, finely chopped	50g	–	–	–
½ tsp. salt	2.5g	–	–	–
½ tsp. Worcestershire sauce	2.5g	–	–	–

Preparation: Mix all ingredients well and let cool. Serve with green salad or vegetable salads.

Yielding: 1³/₄ cups
Calories: 405
Exchange Value: 2 tbsp. = ½ fat exchange
                              = 29 calories

Onion Dressing

Ingredients:	Wt.	C	P	F
1 tbsp. instant minced onion	15g	–	–	–
2 tsp. instant beef broth powder or liquid base	10g	–	–	–
1 tbsp. vinegar	15g	–	–	–
1 tbsp. water	12g	–	–	–
1 tsp. sugar	5g	5	.6	–
1/2 cup dairy sour cream	120g	–	–	20

Preparation: Mix all ingredients well. Refrigerate at least 15 minutes before using. Shake sauce before serving.

Yielding: 3/4 cup
Calories: 202
**Exchange
Value:**   1 1/2 tbsp. = 1/2 fat exchange
                 = 25 calories

Orange Sauce

Ingredients:	Wt.	C	P	F
2¹/₂ tbsp. flour	18g	15	2	—
2 tbsp. sugar	30g	30	4	—
¹/₂ tsp. dry mustard	2.5g	—	—	—
¹/₂ tsp. salt	2.5g	—	—	—
1 cup unsweetened orange juice	200g	20	2	—
2 egg yolks, well beaten	34g	—	6	10
¹/₄ cup lemon juice	50g	5	.5	—

Preparation: Mix flour, sugar, mustard and salt well. Add orange juice and egg yolks. Cook in double boiler, over very hot water (not boiling), stirring constantly, until sauce thickens. Stir in lemon juice; remove from heat and refrigerate.

Yielding: 1¹/₂ cups
Calories: 428
Exchange Value: 2 tbsp. = ¹/₂ bread exchange
= 36 calories

Parisienne Sauce

Ingredients:	Wt.	C	P	F
3/4 cup vinegar	180g	—	—	—
1/2 cup water	100g	—	—	—
1 small scallion, minced	20g	—	—	—
2 tsp. sugar	10g	10	1.3	—
1 tsp. paprika	5g	—	—	—
2 tsp. Worcestershire sauce	10g	—	—	—
1/2 tsp. salt	2.5g	—	—	—
1/2 tsp. celery salt	2.5g	—	—	—
1/4 tsp. dry mustard	—	—	—	—
dash pepper	—	—	—	—

Preparation: Combine all ingredients in a jar with a lid. Cover and shake strenuously before using.

Yielding: 1 1/2 cups
Calories: 45
Exchange Value:
2 tbsp. = free food
= 4 calories

Pinkish Sauce

Ingredients:	Wt.	C	P	F
1 can (10½ ounces) tomato soup, undiluted	300g	45	6	7.5
1 cup vinegar	240g	–	–	–
1½ tsp. Worcestershire sauce	7.5g	–	–	–
2 tbsp. sugar	30g	30	4	–
½ small scallion, minced	10g	–	–	–
2 tsp. dry mustard	10g	–	–	–
1½ tsp. salt	7.5g	–	–	–
½ tsp. paprika	2.5g	–	–	–
¼ tsp. garlic powder	–	–	–	–

Preparation: In a container with a lid, combine all ingredients. Cover and shake thoroughly. Refrigerate.

Yielding: 2¼ cups
Calories: 408
Exchange Value: 2 tbsp. = 1 5% vegetable exchange
= 23 calories

Polynesian Sauce

Ingredients:	Wt.	C	P	F
1 tbsp. cornstarch	8g	7.5	1	–
1 tbsp. sugar	15g	15	2	–
1/2 tsp. curry powder	2.5g	–	–	–
1/2 tsp. paprika	2.5g	–	–	–
1/4 tsp. salt	–	–	–	–
3/4 cup unsweetened pineapple juice	160g	20	2	–
1/4 cup water	50g	–	–	–
1/4 cup catsup	60g	17	2	–
1 tbsp. vinegar	15g	–	–	–

Preparation: In a small saucepan, combine cornstarch, sugar, curry powder, paprika and salt. Gradually, stir in pineapple juice and water. Cook over low heat, stirring constantly, until sauce thickens and bubbles; cook, stirring constantly, for another 1 minute. Remove from heat; add catsup and vinegar. Refrigerate. Serve over main-dish salads.

Yielding: 1 1/4 cups
Calories: 266
Exchange Value: 2 tbsp. = 1 5% vegetable exchange
= 27 calories

Roquefort Cheese Sauce

Ingredients:	Wt.	C	P	F
3 ounces or 6 tbsp. dietetic mayonnaise	90g	–	–	10
1/2 cup light cream (15%)	120g	–	–	20
1 tsp. fresh lemon juice	4g	–	–	–
2 ounces Roquefort cheese, crumbled	60g	–	14	10

Preparation: Mix all ingredients well and refrigerate. Serve with lettuce or with tomato slices or quarters.

Yielding: 1 1/8 cups
Calories: 416
Exchange Value: 2 tbsp. = 1 fat exchange
= 46 calories

Russian Sauce

Ingredients:	Wt.	C	P	F
1 garlic clove, halved	–	–	–	–
3 ounces or 6 tbsp. dietetic mayonnaise	90g	–	–	10
2 tbsp. light cream (15%)	30g	–	–	5
2 tbsp. chili sauce	30g	.5	1	–
15 green olives (stuffed with pimiento), chopped	135g	–	–	15
1 hard-cooked egg, finely chopped	50g	–	7	5
1/2 tsp. salt	2.5g	–	–	–
1/2 tsp. paprika	2.5g	–	–	–

Preparation: Rub garlic halves inside small bowl and throw away. In this small bowl, beat mayonnaise with cream and chili sauce; add remaining ingredients. Stir gently and refrigerate.

Yielding: 1 cup
Calories: 381
Exchange Value: 2 tbsp. = 1 fat exchange
= 48 calories

Sharp Sauce

Ingredients:	Wt.	C	P	F
1/4 cup water	50g	–	–	–
5 tbsp. vinegar	75g	–	–	–
1 tbsp. sugar	15g	15	2	–
2 tsp. cornstarch	5g	5	.6	–
3 tbsp. cold water	38g	–	–	–
1/4 tsp. onion powder	–	–	–	–
1/4 tsp. dry mustard	–	–	–	–
1 tsp. onion seeds	5g	–	–	–
1/4 tsp. paprika	–	–	–	–
1/2 tsp. salt	2.5g	–	–	–
dash pepper	–	–	–	–

Preparation: In a small saucepan, bring 1/4 cup water, vinegar and sugar to boiling point. Remove from heat and add cornstarch, well diluted in cold water. Cook over low heat, stirring constantly, until mixture begins to boil. Remove from heat; add remaining ingredients and beat until smooth. Refrigerate.

Yielding: 3/4 cup
Calories: 90
Exchange Value: 2 tbsp. = 1/2 5% vegetable exchange
                                        or
                          free food if taken in this proportion
                       = 15 calories

Sour Cream Sauce

Ingredients:	Wt.	C	P	F
1 cup dairy sour cream	240g	–	–	40
2 tbsp. white vinegar	30g	–	–	–
non-caloric liquid sweetener to equal 2 tbsp. sugar	–	–	–	–
1/2 tsp. salt	2.5g	–	–	–

Preparation: Mix together all ingredients until very smooth. Serve mostly with coleslaw or lettuce wedges.

Yielding: 1 cup
Calories: 360
Exchange Value: 2 tbsp. = 1 fat exchange
= 45 calories

Spiced Fruit Sauce

Ingredients:	Wt.	C	P	F
¾ cup dairy sour cream	180g	–	–	30
3 ounces unsweetened apple juice	85g	10	1	–
½ tsp. ground cinnamon	2.5g	–	–	–
¼ tsp. ground nutmeg	–	–	–	–
dash salt	–	–	–	–

Preparation: Combine all ingredients and beat with a mixer until very smooth. Serve very cold with a fruit salad.

Yielding: 1¼ cups
Calories: 314
Exchange Value: 2 tbsp. = ½ fat exchange
= 31 calories

Sweet-Sour Sauce

Ingredients:	Wt.	C	P	F
2 tbsp. lemon juice	25g	2.5	–	–
1 tsp. salt	5g	–	–	–
1/4 tsp. dry mustard	–	–	–	–
1 cup evaporated milk	240g	24	16	20

Preparation: Mix lemon juice, salt and mustard. Slowly, stir in evaporated milk, stirring constantly.

Yielding: 1 cup
Calories: 350
Exchange Value: 2 tbsp. = 1/4 whole milk exchange (2 ounces)
= 44 calories

Thousand Islands Sauce

Ingredients:	Wt.	C	P	F
1/4 cup vinegar	60g	–	–	–
1/4 cup chili sauce	60g	17	2	–
1/2 cup evaporated milk	120g	12	8	10
1 hard-cooked egg, chopped	50g	–	7	5
1/4 green pepper, chopped	15g	–	–	–
1 small scallion, minced	20g	–	–	–
1 small garlic clove	–	–	–	–
salt and pepper to taste	–	–	–	–

Preparation: Mix vinegar with chili sauce. Gradually add this mixture to evaporated milk, using an electric or rotary mixer. Stir in remaining ingredients. Refrigerate. Before serving, remove clove garlic. Delicious with green salad.

Yielding: 1 1/4 cups
Calories: 319
Exchange Value: 2 tbsp. = 1/4 fat exchange +
1/4 skim milk exchange (2 ounces)
= 32 calories

Tomato Juice Sauce

Ingredients:	Wt.	C	P	F
1 cup tomato juice	220g	10	1	–
2 tsp. cornstarch	5g	5	.6	–
1 tbsp. lemon juice	12g	–	–	–
1 tsp. Worcestershire sauce	5g	–	–	–
1 garlic clove, mashed	–	–	–	–
1/2 tsp. salt	2.5g	–	–	–
dash pepper	–	–	–	–
minced parsley, to taste	–	–	–	–

Preparation: Bring tomato juice to boiling point. Remove from heat and add cornstarch, well diluted in lemon juice. Cook over low heat, stirring constantly, until mixture begins to boil. Remove from heat and add remaining ingredients. Refrigerate. Delicious with green salads.

Yielding: 1 cup
Calories: 66
Exchange Value: 2 tbsp. = free food if taken in this proportion
= 8 calories

Index

Sauces and Salad Dressings

Alphabetical Index